# The Scar Solution

Step-by Step Guide to Fading and Healing

MARTA BOWEN

Disclaimer:

The Scar Solution

By Marta Bowen

# Contents

# Prologue

To all those who carry the stories etched upon their skin, this book is for you. It is dedicated to the individuals who have navigated the often-challenging journey of wound healing, emerging with the physical and emotional resilience to seek understanding and healing. May this guide serve as a beacon of knowledge, offering clarity, demystifying the complex processes that shape scars, and empowering you to make informed decisions about your skin's future. To the dermatologists, plastic surgeons, nurses, and therapists whose dedication to patient care illuminates the path to scar improvement, your expertise and compassion are invaluable. And finally, to my family and friends, whose unwavering support has been the bedrock upon which this endeavour was built, my deepest gratitude. Your belief in the power of knowledge and the pursuit of well-being fuels this journey.

The human body possesses an extraordinary capacity for repair.

When faced with injury, it embarks on a remarkable, intricate process to mend itself, a testament to biological resilience. Yet, this powerful healing mechanism can sometimes leave behind an indelible mark: a scar. For many, scars are more than just physical reminders; they can carry emotional weight, affecting self-confidence and overall well-being.

"The Scar Solution" was conceived from a desire to bridge the gap between the complex science of scar formation and the everyday individual seeking understanding and effective management. We aim to demystify the biological symphony that leads to scar development, from the initial stages of wound healing to the long-term remodelling of tissues. This book is meticulously designed to be a comprehensive yet accessible resource, catering to those who wish to comprehend the "why" behind their scars. We will delve into the anatomy and physiology of the skin, exploring how different types of injuries lead to the diverse array of scar presentations we commonly encounter – the raised, the indented, the widened. Our journey will meticulously dissect the various treatment modalities available, from time-tested topical applications to cutting-edge procedures. Each option will be presented with clarity, detailing its mechanism of action, potential benefits, limitations, and realistic expectations. Our goal is to equip you with the knowledge necessary to engage in informed discussions with healthcare professionals and to proactively participate in your scar management journey.

Scars are an intrinsic part of the human experience, a visible testament to life's challenges and the body's remarkable ability to heal. Whether resulting from surgery, injury, acne, or burns, scars represent a fundamental biological process: wound healing. However, the repair process, while essential for survival, is not always a perfect restoration of the original tissue. Instead, it often results in a visible alteration of the skin's texture, colour, and structure – what we recognize as a scar.

For individuals living with scars, they can range from a minor cosmetic concern to a significant source of distress, impacting self-esteem and quality of life.

Understanding the science behind scar formation is the crucial first step towards effective management and achieving the best possible aesthetic and functional outcomes.

This book, "The Scar Solution," is born from a passion to empower individuals with knowledge about their scars. We aim to demystify the complex biological processes that govern how our skin heals and how scars form.

Within these pages, we will explore the intricate dance of cells, proteins, and growth factors that orchestrate the wound healing cascade.

You will learn about the different types of scars – from the familiar raised appearance of hypertrophic scars and keloids to the indented depressions of atrophic scars, and the tightening effects of contracture scars.

Each type will be clearly explained, with visual aids to help you identify and understand the specific characteristics of your own scar.

Furthermore, "The Scar Solution" will serve as your comprehensive guide to the ever-evolving landscape of scar treatment.

We will meticulously examine a wide spectrum of interventions, ranging from over-the-counter remedies and silicone-based therapies to advanced dermatological and surgical procedures.

Each treatment option will be presented with a clear explanation of its underlying principles, its efficacy, potential side effects, and what results you can realistically expect.

By providing this detailed information, we aim to equip you with the confidence to discuss treatment options with your healthcare providers and to make informed decisions that align with your personal goals and circumstances.

Our ultimate objective is to foster a sense of hope and control, transforming the often-overwhelming experience of living with scars into a proactive journey toward their successful management.

# CHAPTER ONE
## Identifying Your Scar: A Visual Guide to Types

Hypertrophic scars are thick, raised scars that form as the skin heals.

While they stick out, they always stay within the borders of the original cut or injury. Think of them like a brick wall that was built a few layers too high, but still sits exactly on its original foundation.

They happen because the body gets a bit too enthusiastic and produces extra collagen to quickly patch a wound.

Even though the body overdoes it, the scar doesn't spread to the surrounding healthy skin.

These scars happen because your body's healing process gets out of balance.

Normally, when you have a cut, your body rushes to build a "patch" of collagen.

Once the wound is closed, the body usually tidies up by breaking down the extra material and smoothing things out.

With a hypertrophic scar, that cleanup crew doesn't do its job properly. The cells making the collagen stay "turned on" for too long, or the body fails to clear away the excess.

The result is a pile-up of collagen that makes the scar thick and bumpy. This "over-healing" can be triggered by things like skin tension, an old infection, or simply your genetics.

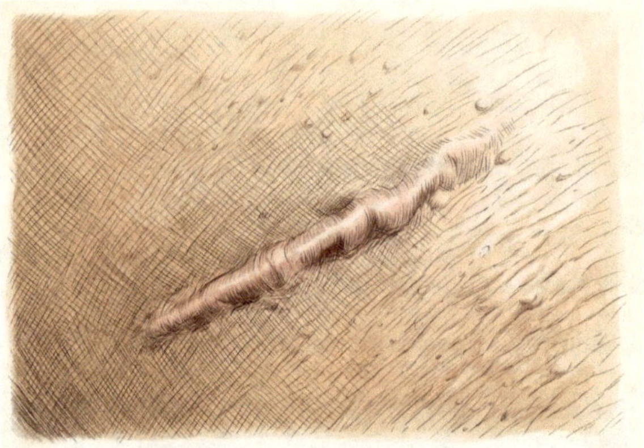

Hypertrophic Scar

You can easily spot a hypertrophic scar by a few key signs.

First, it is raised and bumpy. Instead of lying flat, it sticks up above the rest of your skin. This can range from a tiny bump to a much thicker ridge.

Second, these scars are usually pink or reddish. This colour is a sign that the area still has a lot of blood flow and is actively trying to heal. Over time, the redness usually fades, but it might turn purple or a darker shade before it eventually pales out. The texture of a hypertrophic scar is typically firm and rubbery to the touch. This firmness is a direct result of the dense, organized, albeit excessive, collagen matrix. Unlike the pliable and softer texture of a mature, well-healed scar, a hypertrophic scar often feels dense and slightly raised, creating a distinct textural difference compared to the surrounding epidermis.

Besides being raised, these scars are often very itchy.

This itching happens because the scar tissue has extra nerve endings and is still slightly inflamed.

It can get even worse if the area gets too hot, rubs against certain fabrics, or even when you're feeling stressed.

While they don't usually cause sharp pain, they can feel tender or uncomfortable, especially if they are in a spot where your clothes constantly rub against them.

Hypertrophic scars are very common and can show up after almost any skin injury.

Burns are one of the most frequent causes because the deep damage triggers a massive healing response. Surgery is another big one—the way a cut is stitched, how long it is, and how your body naturally heals all matter.

Even small medical procedures or accidental cuts can lead to these thick scars.

Where the injury happens is also a huge factor. You are much more likely to get one on parts of your body that move or stretch a lot, like your chest, shoulders, upper back, or joints. For example, a scar on your knee or across your chest is more likely to become raised than one on a flatter, stiller area.

To illustrate further, consider a patient who undergoes a knee replacement surgery. The large incision made to access the knee joint is under considerable tension as the leg bends and straightens.

If this tension is not adequately managed during the healing process, the fibroblasts may go into overdrive, laying down excessive collagen to reinforce the wound.

The resulting scar will likely be a raised, firm, and reddish band running along the incision line, confined to the skin that was originally cut, but significantly elevated. Similarly, a severe scald on the forearm can result in a widespread, raised area of scar tissue that follows the contours of the burn, but does not extend beyond the original burned area.

The main difference is that this type of scar stays in its lane. It is defined by the fact that it stays exactly where the original injury was and doesn't spread to the healthy skin around it.

In some instances, hypertrophic scars can appear as thickened, linear bands. Imagine a keloid scar, but crucially, this band stops precisely where the original wound ended. It doesn't spill over or grow beyond these original confines. The surface might be smooth or slightly irregular, and the colour can vary from bright red to a paler pink, depending on the age of the scar and the individual's skin type. The thickness and prominence can also differ greatly. Some may be barely noticeable elevations, while others can be several millimetres in height, casting a distinct shadow when light hits them at an angle. The feeling of tightness associated with hypertrophic scars can also be significant, especially if they traverse over joints, potentially limiting range of motion. This tightness arises from the dense, inelastic nature of the excessive collagen.

Identifying a hypertrophic scar often involves a visual assessment and palpation. If you notice a scar that is raised above the surrounding skin, feels firm, and appears red or pink, especially if it has formed within the last year or two, it is highly likely to be a hypertrophic scar. Crucially, examine its borders. Does it extend beyond the original injury site? If the answer is no, and it remains within the boundaries of the initial wound, then it fits the description of a hypertrophic scar.

If, however, it appears to be growing or extending beyond these original lines, it may be something else, such as a keloid scar, which we will discuss later. The location also provides a clue; scars on the chest, shoulders, or back are statistically more prone to becoming hypertrophic.

When should one seek professional advice regarding a hypertrophic scar? The first indication is if the scar is causing significant cosmetic concern. While hypertrophic scars are generally not dangerous, their appearance can be distressing for some individuals. Secondly, if the scar is causing functional limitations, such as restricting movement due to tightness over a joint, it warrants medical attention. Pain or persistent itching that is not alleviated by over-the-counter remedies is another reason to consult a healthcare professional. Early intervention can sometimes lead to better outcomes, so it is advisable to seek advice from a dermatologist or plastic surgeon if you have concerns about a raised scar, particularly within the first few months to a year of its formation.

They can accurately diagnose the scar type and discuss potential management strategies. Understanding whether you have a hypertrophic scar is the first step in effectively managing its appearance and any associated symptoms.

While hypertrophic scars are like a garden bed that grows a bit too high but stays in its place, keloids are like an invasive vine that crawls everywhere.

The big difference is that keloids don't stop at the edges of the original cut; they spread out and take over the healthy skin around them.

They are the "overachievers" of the scar world because the body's healing process goes into overdrive and doesn't know when to quit, creating a scar that is much larger than the initial injury.

he main thing to know about a keloid is that it doesn't know when to stop.

Unlike other scars that stay put, a keloid spreads out and grows much larger and thicker than the original cut. This happens because the cells that make the "patch" (collagen) ignore the signal to quit. They keep working for months or even years, piling up extra material in a messy, disorganized way.

The result is a raised, thick, and sometimes discoloured bump that actively invades the healthy skin around it.

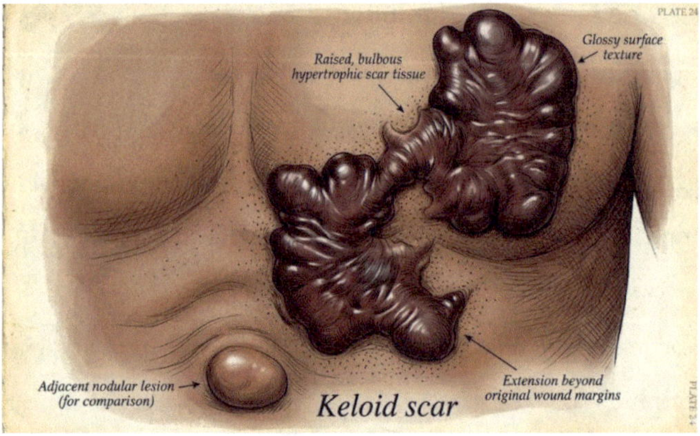


Visually, keloids present a distinct and often alarming appearance. They are typically raised, often significantly so, and can vary in colour from pink and red to darker, purplish or brown hues, particularly in individuals with darker skin tones.

The surface of a keloid can feel firm and rubbery, but also irregular and nodular.

Unlike the relatively smooth surface of a mature hypertrophic scar, keloids can have a lumpy, bumpy texture. Their size is a key differentiator; while hypertrophic scars are generally limited to the dimensions of the original wound, keloids can be several centimetres in diameter, dwarfing the initial injury.

Some keloids may even develop claw-like extensions that creep beyond the original wound margins, further emphasizing their invasive nature. The borders of a keloid are often ill-defined as they spread, creating a more amorphous and spreading shape compared to the sharply demarcated edges of a contained hypertrophic scar.

The location of the original injury plays a significant role in the propensity for keloid formation. Certain areas of the body are more prone to developing keloids due to inherent tension or susceptibility. The chest, shoulders, upper back, earlobes (especially from piercings), and the sternal area are classic sites for keloid development.

This predisposition is thought to be related to the skin's elasticity and the forces it experiences in these regions during the healing process. However, keloids can form anywhere on the body, from minor nicks and scratches to more significant burns and surgical incisions. Even seemingly insignificant injuries like insect bites or acne lesions can, in susceptible individuals, result in the formation of a keloid.

Beyond the visual presentation, keloid scars can be accompanied by a range of uncomfortable symptoms.

Persistent itching (pruritus) is a common complaint, and it can be intense and deeply bothersome, interfering with sleep and daily activities.

The itching is likely due to the increased density of nerve endings within the keloid tissue and the ongoing inflammatory processes. Some individuals also experience pain or tenderness, particularly when the keloid is touched or subjected to pressure. This discomfort can range from a dull ache to sharp, shooting pains.

In some cases, keloids can also cause a sensation of tightness, especially if they are located over joints, potentially leading to restricted movement and functional impairment. This tightness arises from the dense, inelastic nature of the excessive collagen.

A particularly noteworthy aspect of keloid scars is their disproportionate prevalence in certain populations. Individuals with darker skin tones, particularly those of African, Asian, and Hispanic descent, have a significantly higher incidence of keloid formation compared to individuals with lighter skin. This suggests a genetic predisposition and a heightened inflammatory response in these individuals that makes them more susceptible to this aggressive form of scarring. While the exact genetic mechanisms are still being investigated, it is understood that there are likely multiple genes involved that influence fibroblast activity and collagen synthesis. Family history also plays a role; if you have close relatives who develop keloids, your own risk is elevated. This genetic component underscores the importance of understanding an individual's personal and familial history when assessing scar risk.

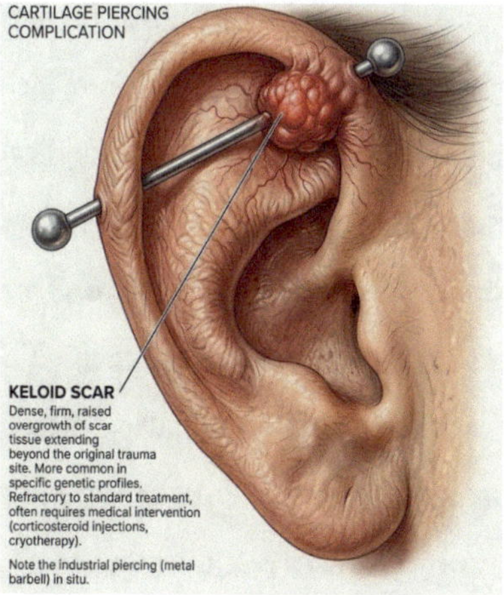


To further illustrate the aggressive nature of keloids, consider the case of a minor earlobe piercing. In most individuals, this results in a small, well-healed puncture. However, in someone predisposed to keloids, the small wound can become the site of an unsightly, raised, rubbery mass that grows to encompass the entire earlobe and even extend onto the cheek. Similarly, a small surgical scar on the chest, perhaps from a biopsy, might in a keloid-prone individual transform into a large, thick, and spreading keloid that far exceeds the original incision in size and prominence. These examples highlight the critical difference: keloids do not respect the boundaries of the original wound; they actively invade and expand.

It is essential to tell the difference between these two types of scars because they are treated differently.

The main thing to look for is the boundary: Hypertrophic scars stay exactly where you were hurt. If you can only see the raised part where the cut was, it's likely this type. Keloid scars grow past the original injury and take over the healthy skin nearby. Their timelines also differ:

Hypertrophic scars usually show up within a few weeks or months and often get better or flatter on their own over time. Keloids can keep growing for years and rarely go away without medical help.

The invasive nature of keloids can lead to significant cosmetic and psychological distress for individuals. Their prominent appearance can draw unwanted attention and impact self-esteem. The itching and pain associated with keloids can also be debilitating. Because keloids are so persistent and prone to recurrence, management often requires a multidisciplinary approach and a commitment to ongoing treatment.

This is where understanding the unique characteristics of keloids becomes paramount. Unlike hypertrophic scars, which may respond favourably to less intensive interventions, keloids often necessitate more aggressive and sustained therapeutic strategies to control their growth and alleviate symptoms.

A keloid forms because your body's healing system gets stuck in "attack mode" and doesn't know when to quit. Normally, your body goes through three steps: it clears out the mess, builds a patch of collagen, and then tidies everything up. With a keloid, the middle step goes haywire. The "building" cells stay active for way too long, piling up extra collagen in a messy, unorganized heap. At the same time, the body's "cleanup crew" fails to break down the extra material. This is often caused by a chemical imbalance in the skin—specifically a growth factor called TGF-beta—that tells the cells to keep overproducing. The result is a thick, tough scar that just keeps growing.

The clinical presentation of keloids can vary widely, adding another layer of complexity to their identification. While the classic keloid is a raised, firm, and often irregular mass extending beyond the original wound, there are variations. Some keloids may present as multiple small nodules, especially following conditions like acne or folliculitis. Others can be larger, flattened plaques that spread outwards. The term "keloid" is derived from the Greek word "chele," meaning claw, aptly describing the tendency of some keloids to develop pseudopods or finger-like projections that extend beyond the initial wound margin.

The colour of a keloid can also be an indicator of its activity.

While newer keloids are often erythematous due to increased vascularity, older, more mature keloids may become hypopigmented (lighter than the surrounding skin) or hyperpigmented (darker than the surrounding skin), depending on the individual's skin type and the ongoing biological processes within the scar. Keloids can cause severe itching and pain that significantly affect daily life.

The itching is often intense and frequently gets worse at night, which can make it hard to sleep. It can be triggered by simple things like heat, your clothes rubbing against the scar, or even feeling stressed. The pain can feel like burning, stinging, or sharp shooting sensations. This happens because the nerves inside the scar tissue are damaged or extra sensitive. These symptoms are often worse if the keloid is in a spot that gets bumped or pressed a lot. Beyond the physical symptoms, keloids can take a heavy emotional toll. Because they are often large and noticeable, they can make people feel very self-conscious, leading to anxiety, depression, or a desire to hide the scars and avoid social situations

Understanding the genetic and ethnic predispositions to keloid formation is vital for both patients and clinicians. Individuals with a family history of keloids or those belonging to ethnic groups with a higher prevalence should be made aware of the increased risk following any skin injury. This awareness allows for proactive discussions about scar prevention and early intervention strategies. For instance, if a patient with a known predisposition requires surgery, meticulous surgical technique and close post-operative monitoring can be employed to minimize the risk of keloid development.

Similarly, procedures like earlobe piercings in individuals with a history of keloids should be approached with extreme caution and often managed with prophylactic treatments. The role of genetics is complex, involving multiple genes that influence immune responses, fibroblast behaviour, and collagen metabolism. Research is ongoing to identify specific genetic markers that could predict an individual's risk of developing keloids, which would pave the way for more personalized prevention and treatment strategies.

The distinction between keloid and hypertrophic scars is not merely academic; it has profound implications for treatment. Hypertrophic scars, being contained within the wound borders, often respond well to a range of therapies including silicone sheeting, pressure therapy, and topical corticosteroid injections. Keloids, with their aggressive extra-lesional growth, frequently require more intensive and multimodal approaches. Surgical excision alone is often insufficient and can lead to recurrence, sometimes even larger than the original keloid. Therefore, treatment plans for keloids often involve a combination of therapies. For example, surgical excision may be followed by radiation therapy, corticosteroid injections, or the application of silicone gel sheeting and pressure dressings to minimize the chance of recurrence. Understanding the overachieving nature of keloid collagen production is the first step in appreciating why these scars demand a more persistent and often aggressive management strategy.

They are a testament to the body's complex and sometimes unpredictable healing mechanisms, requiring a nuanced and patient-centred approach to achieve the best possible outcomes.

In contrast to the raised and often exuberant collagen production seen in hypertrophic and keloid scars, atrophic scars present a fundamentally different challenge to the skin's surface. Instead of rising above, these scars are characterized by a noticeable indentation or depression, creating a sunken appearance.

This loss of dermal volume is the hallmark of atrophic scarring, and it stems from a deficiency in tissue regeneration or an insufficient deposition of collagen during the healing process. While raised scars are a testament to an overactive healing response, atrophic scars signify a healing process that has fallen short, leaving behind a void where healthy, plump tissue once resided.

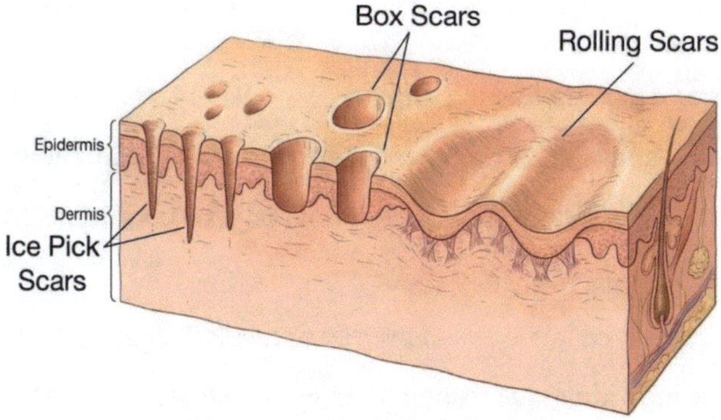


**Plate 14: Common Types of Atrophic Acne Scarring**
Key: Ice Pick Scars, b. - Box Scars, or Boxcar Scars, ծ. - Rolling Scars

Atrophic scars are basically the opposite of raised scars—they look like dents or pits in the skin.

They happen when an injury or illness destroys collagen and the body doesn't fully "fill in the hole" during the healing process.

The two most common causes are:

Acne: Especially deep or painful pimples (like cysts). The inflammation eats away at the skin's support, and when the pimple heals, it leaves a sunken spot behind.

Chickenpox: The blisters from this virus can damage the deeper layers of skin. When they scab over and heal, they often leave behind small, pitted scars.

In both cases, the skin loses its underlying structure, resulting in a depression rather than a smooth surface.

Major weight changes can also cause these "sunken" or indented scars.

When you gain weight quickly, your skin stretches, pulling on the collagen and elastic fibers that keep it firm. If you then lose weight rapidly—like after weight-loss surgery or a strict diet—your skin might not snap back into place.

This leaves the skin looking thin, loose, or dented, especially on the belly, thighs, and butt. Because you've also lost the fat underneath that used to "fill out" the skin, these depressions and scars become much more obvious.

Furthermore, certain types of injuries or medical conditions can predispose individuals to atrophic scarring. Traumatic injuries that involve significant tissue loss, such as deep cuts or abrasions that go beyond the superficial epidermis and into the dermis, may heal with an atrophic component if the repair process is inadequate.

Certain autoimmune conditions that affect connective tissue can also contribute to the breakdown of dermal structures, potentially leading to atrophic scarring.

The key underlying mechanism, regardless of the inciting event, is a deficit in the dermal matrix – the structural framework that gives skin its firmness and smoothness.

The visual characteristics of atrophic scars can vary significantly, and dermatologists and plastic surgeons have developed specific terminology to describe these different presentations. This classification is crucial not only for accurate diagnosis but also for guiding treatment strategies, as each type of atrophic scar responds best to particular interventions. The most common categories of atrophic scars are ice pick scars, boxcar scars, and rolling scars. Understanding the nuances of each type allows for a more precise approach to improving the skin's texture and appearance.

Ice pick scars are perhaps the most challenging type of atrophic scar to treat. They are named for their resemblance to punctures made by an ice pick, appearing as narrow, deep fissures that extend into the dermis. These scars are typically very small in diameter, often less than 2 millimetres, but their depth is their defining feature. Visually, they create a pitted appearance on the skin's surface, making it look as though tiny holes have been punched into it. The edges of an ice pick scar are often sharply defined, and the scar can appear to be a narrow tunnel rather than a broad depression. Because they are so deep and narrow, they are notoriously difficult to fill in from below. The underlying tissue loss is concentrated at a focal point, making it hard for the body to naturally regenerate sufficient collagen to bring the base of the scar level with the surrounding skin. In individuals with lighter skin tones, these scars may appear as small, white, or flesh-coloured depressions.

In those with darker skin tones, they can sometimes be more noticeable due to slight post-inflammatory hyperpigmentation or hypopigmentation around the edges. Their prevalence is highest on the cheeks and forehead, areas particularly prone to severe acne. The process of their formation involves a deep follicular inflammation that destroys the surrounding collagen and elastin, leading to a collapse of the overlying epidermis. The scar is essentially a remnant of this collapsed follicular structure, leaving a deep, narrow void. The appearance can be quite distressing, as even a small number of these scars can significantly disrupt the overall smoothness of the skin, especially in areas where light can catch the subtle depressions.

Boxcar scars are another common form of atrophic scarring, often associated with acne. Unlike the narrow, pointed nature of ice pick scars, boxcar scars are wider and more U-shaped depressions with sharply defined vertical edges. They are reminiscent of the shape of a box or a crater. These scars are typically larger in diameter than ice pick scars, ranging from 1 to 4 millimetres, and they extend down into the dermis. The depth can vary, but they generally do not reach the deepest layers of the skin. The defining characteristic is their "punched out" appearance, with steep, almost perpendicular sides. This contrasts with the sloping or irregular edges seen in some other types of scarring. Boxcar scars can appear on the cheeks, temples, and forehead. They are often the result of inflammatory lesions, such as papules or pustules, that heal with a loss of collagen, causing the overlying epidermis to sag. The distinct, sharp edges are a consequence of the way the skin collapses inward after the inflammatory process has subsided.

The wider base means that there is more surface area affected, and the loss of dermal volume is more pronounced than in an ice pick scar. This type of scar can make the skin appear uneven and textured, particularly when viewed in profile or under certain lighting conditions. While they are not as deep as ice pick scars, their width can make them quite noticeable and contribute to a generally rougher skin texture.

Rolling scars are characterized by their undulating or wave-like appearance across the skin's surface. These scars are caused by fibrous bands of tissue that form beneath the skin, tethering the epidermis down to the deeper subcutaneous tissue. This pulling creates a rolling or uneven topography, giving the skin a wavy, depressed look. Unlike boxcar or ice pick scars, which have distinct edges, rolling scars have broader, shallower depressions with sloping sides and ill-defined borders. They are typically larger than the other types of atrophic scars, sometimes extending over several millimetres. The characteristic "rolling" appearance is a result of the varying depths of these depressions, creating a landscape of hills and valleys across the affected area, often the cheeks. This type of scarring is a consequence of the body's attempt to repair deeper damage, but instead of filling the void, it creates fibrotic bands that pull the overlying skin downwards. The skin between these bands appears normal or slightly raised, while the skin over the bands is depressed, leading to the characteristic undulating pattern. The overall impression is one of a loss of smoothness and firmness in the skin's texture. The fibrous septa responsible for rolling scars can be challenging to break down, as they are deeply embedded within the dermal and subcutaneous layers.

It is important to differentiate atrophic scars from other types of skin irregularities. For instance, enlarged pores, which can appear as small, dark spots, are often confused with ice pick scars. However, enlarged pores are simply dilated hair follicles and do not represent a loss of dermal tissue.

Similarly, mild post-inflammatory hyperpigmentation or hypopigmentation can create temporary colour changes that might be mistaken for scars, but these are superficial discolorations that lack the textural defect of true atrophic scarring. The absence of dermal volume is the defining characteristic that separates atrophic scars from these other conditions.

When assessing a scar, one should look for a depression, a sunken quality, and a loss of the normal smooth contour of the skin.

The way sunken scars form depends on how much damage was done deep inside your skin.

Using acne as an example, when a deep pimple "pops" under the skin, it releases chemicals that actually dissolve your natural collagen.

Your body tries to fix the damage, but sometimes it just can't build back enough "filler" to level the surface. This leaves a hollow spot or a dent.

The shape of the scar depends on how deep the original breakout was:

Boxcar or Rolling scars: These are usually shallower and wider, caused by surface-level inflammation.

Ice pick scars: These look like tiny, deep holes made by a needle, usually caused by very deep infections that destroyed a lot of tissue in one spot.

In the context of chickenpox, the viral infection causes vesicles (blisters) that, when scratched or infected, can penetrate into the dermis. The healing of these lesions involves the formation of granulation tissue, which is then replaced by fibrous scar tissue. If the underlying tissue damage is substantial, or if the inflammatory response is excessive, the resulting scar tissue may be less organized and contain less collagen than the surrounding healthy skin. This can lead to a depression or pit in the skin's surface. The size and depth of the chickenpox lesion, as well as any secondary trauma or infection, will influence the severity and type of atrophic scar that develops.

The process of significant weight loss also contributes to atrophic scarring through different mechanisms. As fat cells (adipocytes) in the subcutaneous tissue shrink, the overlying skin loses its underlying support.

This can cause the skin to appear looser and thinner. If the skin has been stretched for a prolonged period, the collagen and elastin fibres within the dermis may become permanently damaged and lose their elasticity. When the weight is lost, these weakened fibres cannot snap back into place, leading to a degree of laxity and subtle depressions, particularly where the loss of volume is most pronounced.

This is distinct from the direct tissue destruction seen in acne or chickenpox, but the end result is a visually noticeable loss of dermal volume.

Understanding these underlying mechanisms is crucial for effective treatment.

Atrophic scars represent a deficit, a lack of tissue volume.

Therefore, treatments aim to either stimulate the body to produce more collagen, to physically break down the fibrous bands that tether the skin down, or to resurface the skin to minimize the visibility of the indentations. This often involves a multi-pronged approach. For instance, treatments like microneedling, fractional laser resurfacing, and chemical peels work by creating controlled injury to the skin, which triggers the body's natural wound healing response, leading to increased collagen production and dermal remodelling. Dermal fillers can be used to directly plump up the depressed areas, temporarily filling the void. Surgical techniques, such as succession, are specifically designed to break the fibrous bands responsible for rolling scars, allowing the skin to lift. Punch excision is a technique where individual ice pick scars are surgically removed and the resulting small wound is closed with sutures, often resulting in a less noticeable, linear scar.

The visual identification of atrophic scars is a key step in developing a personalized treatment plan. A thorough examination by a dermatologist or plastic surgeon, often under magnification and with specialized lighting, is necessary to accurately assess the type, depth, and distribution of atrophic scarring. This allows for the selection of the most appropriate and effective therapeutic modalities, aiming to restore a smoother, more even skin texture and to improve the overall aesthetic appearance. The sunken nature, the loss of dermal volume, and the specific morphology – whether pitted, crater-like, or undulating – are the key features that dermatologists look for when diagnosing and categorizing atrophic scars.

This detailed visual understanding is the foundation upon which successful scar revision strategies are built.

Contracture scars represent a distinct and often challenging category of scarring, characterized primarily by their significant tightening effect on the skin. Unlike the raised exuberance of hypertrophic scars or the subtle depressions of atrophic scars, contracture scars are defined by a palpable and often visible restriction of movement. This tightening is a direct consequence of the dense, fibrous scar tissue that forms during the healing process, particularly after severe injuries such as burns or deep lacerations. This scar tissue doesn't simply lie on the surface; it actively pulls the edges of the wound together, often with such force that it can compromise the underlying structures, including muscles, tendons, and nerves. The visual appearance of a contracture scar is typically one of smooth, shiny, and remarkably tight bands of tissue. This tautness can lead to a distorted appearance of the skin, making it seem almost stretched and less pliable than healthy skin.

**PLATE 42: CICATRICIAL CONTRACTURE SCAR**

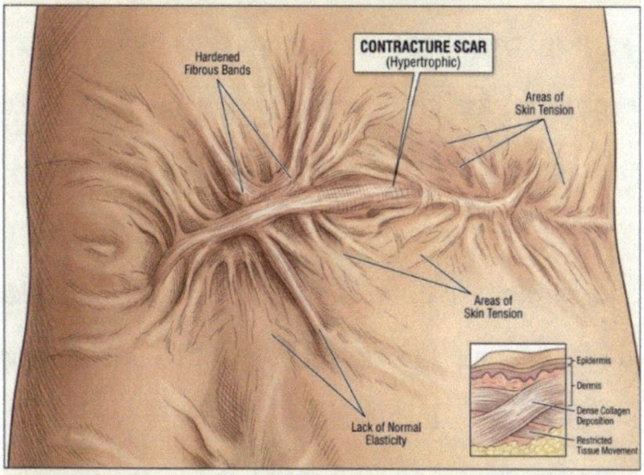


A severe cicatricial contracture scar on the skin surface, exhibiting characteristic raised, multi-directional fibrous bands that restrict movement. Note the high tension and poor extensibility of the tissue, frequently following severe burn or deep dermal trauma.

Contracture scars happen when your body overreacts while healing a major injury. After a deep wound—like a severe burn—your body rushes to close the gap. Instead of a normal scar, it builds thick, tough bands of stiff collagen. As this scar matures, it acts like a tight drawstring, pulling the healthy skin around it inward and making the area feel extremely tight.

This tightening doesn't happen all at once; it can keep pulling for weeks or even months. The deeper the injury, the stronger these bands become, which is why they can eventually make it hard to move that part of your body.

The functional implications of contracture scars can be profound and significantly impact a person's quality of life. When a contracture scar forms across a joint – such as the elbow, knee, fingers, or neck – the tightening of the skin can severely limit the range of motion. Imagine a person with a burn contracture across their elbow. The scar tissue may pull the skin so tightly that they are unable to fully extend their arm, making everyday activities like reaching for an object, dressing, or even performing basic hygiene incredibly difficult. Similarly, contracture scars on the hands can impede the ability to grasp, hold, or perform fine motor tasks. Those forming around the neck can restrict head movement, impacting vision and the ability to swallow or speak comfortably. This loss of mobility is not just a physical inconvenience; it can lead to psychological distress, social isolation, and a significant decrease in independence. The tightness can also be accompanied by discomfort or pain, especially when attempting to stretch the affected area. Nerves caught within the scar tissue can become compressed, leading to numbness, tingling, or chronic pain.

Blood flow can also be compromised, potentially leading to a bluish or cool appearance of the affected limb.

The cosmetic concerns associated with contracture scars are also considerable. Beyond the functional limitations, the appearance of these scars can be a source of significant self-consciousness. The smooth, shiny, and often discoloured nature of the scar tissue, combined with the distortion it can cause to the surrounding skin and features, can be visually distressing. For instance, a contracture scar across the face, perhaps from an accident or a surgical revision, can alter facial symmetry and expressions, leading to significant aesthetic concerns. The colour of contracture scars can vary. Initially, they may be reddish or purplish due to increased vascularity. As they mature, they can become paler, sometimes appearing almost white or translucent, contrasting sharply with the surrounding skin. This stark contrast, coupled with the tight, drawn appearance, can draw unwanted attention. The texture

is typically smooth, lacking the normal pores and fine lines of healthy skin, contributing to an artificial or unnatural look.

The location of a contracture scar is a critical determinant of its impact. Scars across the palmar surface of the hand or fingers can severely limit flexion and extension.

Those that form on the soles of the feet can make walking painful and difficult. Contractures around the mouth can affect speech and eating.

Any scar that crosses a flexor surface, where skin is naturally creased, is at higher risk of becoming a contracture scar due to the constant stretching and movement in that area.

For example, scars in the antecubital fossa (the bend of the elbow) or the popliteal fossa (the bend of the knee) are particularly prone to developing significant functional impairments.

The development of contracture scars is not always immediate; the process of contraction can continue for many months or even years post-injury, meaning that the functional and cosmetic limitations can worsen over time if not properly managed.

The importance of early assessment and intervention for contracture scars cannot be overstated. Recognizing the potential for tightening and functional impairment soon after the initial injury is crucial. Healthcare professionals, particularly those involved in burn care, trauma management, and reconstructive surgery, are trained to identify the risk factors and to initiate early management strategies. These strategies often begin with meticulous wound care to promote optimal healing and to minimize the extent of scarring. Gentle range-of-motion exercises, often guided by physical or occupational therapists, are initiated as soon as it is medically safe to do so. These exercises aim to keep the joints flexible and to prevent the scar tissue from adhering to underlying structures and limiting movement. Positional therapy, using splints or braces to maintain limbs in an extended or functional position, is also a cornerstone of early management, particularly in burn patients.

This helps to counteract the natural tendency of scar tissue to contract.

The visual identification of contracture scars involves a careful examination of the scar's texture, colour, and its relationship to surrounding anatomical structures, especially joints.

A trained eye will look for signs of tension, such as stretched or thinned skin overlying the scar, distortion of natural skin lines, or the absence of normal skin folds. The practitioner will also assess the scar's impact on skin elasticity by gently trying to pinch or stretch the tissue.

The range of motion of any adjacent joints will be evaluated, noting any limitations or pain experienced by the patient. Palpation of the scar can reveal its depth and the extent to which it is adhering to deeper tissues. The "shiny" appearance is often due to the absence of normal skin appendages like hair follicles and sweat glands, and the flattened, dense nature of the collagen. The tightness can sometimes be so severe that the scar appears almost embedded into the underlying tissue, creating a visible tethering effect.

In summary, contracture scars are a consequence of the body's aggressive healing response to significant trauma, characterized by the formation of dense, fibrous scar tissue that pulls and tightens the skin. This tightening can lead to severe functional limitations, particularly around joints, impacting mobility and daily life.

Aesthetically, they can cause significant distortion and disfigurement. Their smooth, shiny, and taut appearance is a visual hallmark. Given their potential for profound impact on a patient's well-being, early recognition, proactive management, and often specialized surgical or therapeutic interventions are paramount in mitigating the detrimental effects of contracture scars.

Understanding these characteristics is the first step in addressing this challenging form of scarring and working towards restoring both function and appearance.

Stretch marks, medically termed striae distensae, represent a distinct category of skin markings that, while not true scars in the way a surgical incision or a deep wound's aftermath is, are often perceived as such by individuals experiencing them.

Their formation is fundamentally different from the cicatricial process of wound healing. Instead of originating from trauma or injury that breaches the skin's integrity and necessitates a complex repair mechanism, stretch marks arise from a mechanical stretching of the dermis, the skin's middle layer. This stretching causes the collagen and elastin fibers, responsible for the skin's strength and elasticity, to tear. Imagine a balloon being overinflated; eventually, the surface begins to show stress lines. The skin, when subjected to rapid or prolonged stretching beyond its capacity, undergoes a similar phenomenon.

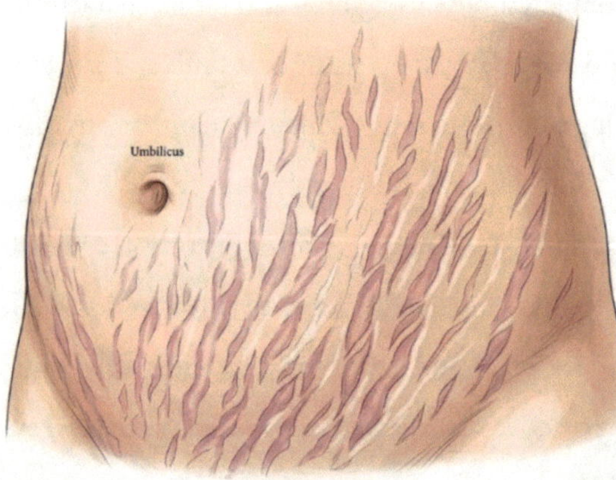


*stretch marks*

Fig. 14a: Close-up view of abdominal striae distensae in an adult female.

The most common culprits behind this excessive stretching are periods of rapid growth or weight fluctuation.

During puberty, adolescents often develop stretch marks as their bodies grow rapidly.

Similarly, pregnancy is a frequent precursor to striae, particularly on the abdomen, breasts, hips, and thighs, as the skin expands to accommodate the growing fetus.

Significant weight gain, whether due to lifestyle, medical conditions, or bodybuilding, can also lead to these dermal tears. Certain hormonal changes, especially those involving corticosteroids, can predispose an individual to stretch marks by weakening the collagen fibres, making them more susceptible to tearing even with moderate stretching. The genetic predisposition also plays a role; if your parents or close relatives have stretch marks, you are more likely to develop them.

Visually, stretch marks typically manifest as linear depressions or streaks on the skin. In their initial stages, often referred to as striae rubrae, they may appear reddish, purplish, or even pink. This coloration is due to increased vascularity and inflammation within the damaged dermal tissue. They can be slightly raised or flat at this point. Over time, as the inflammatory process subsides and the dermal tears begin to heal without complete restoration of the original collagen structure, the colour of the striae begins to change. They gradually fade into a paler, whiter, or silvery hue, becoming what are known as striae albae. This silvery appearance is a hallmark of mature stretch marks, where the blood vessels have constricted, and the tissue has become more fibrotic and less vascularized. At this stage, they are typically depressed below the surrounding skin surface, giving them a slightly indented or atrophic quality. Their texture can feel smoother than the surrounding skin, and they may lack the fine wrinkles or pores characteristic of healthy dermis.

The pattern is usually parallel and can cover significant areas of the body, following the lines of tension and stretching.

Distinguishing stretch marks from true scars is crucial for appropriate understanding and management. Unlike scars, which often arise from a distinct injury event and can vary greatly in thickness, texture, and colour depending on the nature of the wound and the healing response, stretch marks are a consequence of intrinsic dermal disruption due to mechanical stress.

While some scars might be depressed (atrophic), their formation is linked to insufficient collagen production during wound healing.

Stretch marks, on the other hand, are a result of over-stretching leading to fibre breakage.

While both can alter the skin's appearance and texture, the underlying cause and initial presentation differ significantly.

A laceration scar will often follow a specific line of injury, while stretch marks tend to appear in areas of greatest skin tension and expansion.

Beyond stretch marks, another common skin phenomenon that individuals may mistake for scarring involves changes in skin pigmentation following inflammation. These are known as post-inflammatory hyperpigmentation (PIH) and post-inflammatory hypopigmentation.

It is vital to understand that these are not true scars; they are temporary or sometimes persistent alterations in skin colour rather than structural changes to the dermis.

**Post Inflammatory Hyperpigmentation**

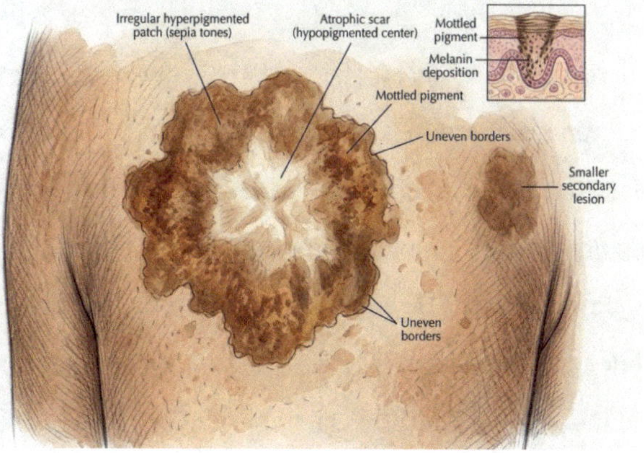


Post-inflammatory hyperpigmentation refers to the darkening of the skin that occurs after an inflammatory process has subsided. This can be triggered by a variety of conditions, including acne, eczema, psoriasis, insect bites, minor injuries, or even certain cosmetic procedures like chemical peels or laser treatments. When the skin experiences inflammation, it triggers a response from melanocytes, the cells responsible for producing melanin, the pigment that gives skin its colour. In response to the inflammation, melanocytes can become overactive, producing an excess amount of melanin. This extra melanin is then deposited in the epidermis and sometimes deeper into the dermis, leading to the formation of dark spots or patches. The severity and duration of the initial inflammation often correlate with the intensity of the hyperpigmentation. For instance, picking at pimples or experiencing severe acne lesions is more likely to result in noticeable PIH than mild, infrequent breakouts.

The appearance of PIH is typically characterized by brown, black, or grey discoloured areas on the skin.

The exact shade can vary depending on an individual's natural skin tone. In individuals with lighter skin, PIH might appear as light brown spots, whereas in those with darker skin tones, it can manifest as deeper brown or even black patches. These areas are usually flat and do not represent a change in skin texture or thickness. The distribution of PIH often mirrors the location of the original inflammatory condition. For example, acne-induced PIH commonly appears on the face, chest, and back, while eczema-related PIH might be found on the areas affected by the rash. Unlike true scars, PIH generally does not cause any alteration in the skin's surface smoothness or elevation. The skin in the affected area retains its normal texture, pore structure, and elasticity. This lack of textural change is a key differentiator.

On the other hand, post-inflammatory hypopigmentation is the opposite effect: a lightening of the skin following inflammation. This occurs when the inflammatory process damages or suppresses the melanocytes in the affected area, leading to a reduction in melanin production. Conditions like eczema, psoriasis, severe burns, or even certain treatments like cryotherapy can sometimes result in hypopigmentation. In some cases, trauma to the skin can physically damage the melanocytes, impairing their ability to produce pigment.

Visually, post-inflammatory hypopigmentation presents as lighter-than-normal patches or spots on the skin. These areas appear paler, sometimes almost white, against the surrounding skin. The contrast is particularly noticeable in individuals with darker skin tones. Like PIH, hypopigmentation typically does not involve any textural changes to the skin.

The affected skin remains smooth and retains its normal feel. The size and shape of the hypopigmented areas can vary widely, depending on the extent and nature of the preceding inflammation or injury. In some instances, the melanocytes may eventually recover their function, and the skin colour can return to normal over time. However, in cases of severe or prolonged inflammation, or where melanocytes have been significantly damaged, the hypopigmentation can be permanent.

When differentiating these post-inflammatory pigmentary changes from actual scars, several visual cues are paramount. The first and most significant is texture. True scars, particularly hypertrophic and atrophic scars, involve a change in the skin's structural composition, leading to alterations in thickness, smoothness, and pliability. Stretch marks, while not a result of wound healing, also represent a physical tear and subsequent healing in the dermis, which can result in a textural difference.

Post-inflammatory hyperpigmentation and hypopigmentation, however, are primarily concerns of colour. The skin in these areas typically feels the same as the surrounding healthy skin. If you gently pinch or stretch the skin in an area of PIH or hypopigmentation, it will behave much like the surrounding skin, unlike a tight contracture scar or the sometimes-rubbery texture of a hypertrophic scar. Another key distinction lies in the timeline and cause. True scars are the direct result of wound healing. Stretch marks are a result of mechanical stretching.

Post-inflammatory pigmentary changes are sequelae of inflammation or injury that affect pigment-producing cells.

If you can recall a specific event of skin injury, deep cut, burn, or surgical procedure, the resulting mark is likely a scar. If the mark appeared after a period of rapid growth, weight change, or pregnancy, it is likely a stretch mark. If the discoloration appeared after an inflammatory skin condition like acne or eczema, or a specific treatment, it is likely post-inflammatory hyper- or hypopigmentation.

To further illustrate, consider an individual who has had severe acne. They might notice persistent dark spots on their cheeks where pimples once were.

These are typically PIH. The skin in these spots feels normal, and there are no raised or depressed areas.

In contrast, if that same individual had a deep cystic acne lesion that eroded into the dermis, the resulting mark might be a small, slightly indented (atrophic) scar, noticeable not just by its colour but by its altered texture and depth.

Similarly, a burn that heals with significant scarring will exhibit textural changes—thickening, tightness, or depressed areas—whereas a mild burn that causes temporary inflammation might result in transient PIH or hypopigmentation, where the skin colour eventually returns to normal without textural alterations.

Understanding these differences is vital for setting realistic expectations regarding treatment.

While true scars often require specific dermatological or surgical interventions to improve their appearance and texture, pigmentary changes are primarily addressed by managing melanin production.

Treatments for PIH, for instance, often focus on exfoliation and inhibiting melanin synthesis, whereas treatments for hypopigmentation might aim to stimulate melanocyte activity or camouflage the affected areas.

Recognizing whether you are dealing with a scar, a stretch mark, or a pigmentary change guides the selection of the most effective therapeutic approach, ensuring that efforts are directed towards the root cause of the skin's altered appearance. This comprehensive visual guide aims to empower you to accurately identify these common skin concerns, differentiating them from more complex scar presentations and paving the way for informed discussions with your healthcare provider.

# CHAPTER TWO

## Understanding Your Scar: The Body's Story of Healing

When our skin, the body's largest organ and primary defence, encounters an injury, whether a simple scrape, a surgical incision, or a more significant trauma, it doesn't simply remain damaged. Instead, an extraordinary, complex, and elegantly orchestrated biological ballet begins.

This intricate process, known as wound healing, is the body's innate and remarkable method for repairing breaches in its protective barrier.

It's a cascade of cellular events, molecular signals, and tissue remodelling designed to restore integrity, prevent infection, and ultimately, to mend the damage.

Understanding this fundamental process is not just an academic exercise; it's the bedrock upon which all our efforts to manage and improve scars are built. Without appreciating the body's natural repair mechanisms, we cannot fully comprehend why scars form, why they look the way they do, or how we can best influence their development for a more favourable outcome. Think of it as understanding the original blueprint and the construction crew's efforts before critiquing the final building.

The wound healing process is not a single event but a continuum that unfolds in distinct, yet overlapping, phases.

While textbooks often divide it into four stages—hemostasis, inflammation, proliferation, and remodelling—for the purpose of understanding scar formation, we can focus on the three primary phases that directly shape the tissue that eventually becomes scar: inflammation, proliferation, and remodelling. Each phase is critical, and the efficiency and balance of these stages profoundly influence the final appearance of the scar. It's a dynamic interplay, where one phase transitions into the next, driven by a symphony of biochemical signals and cellular activities.

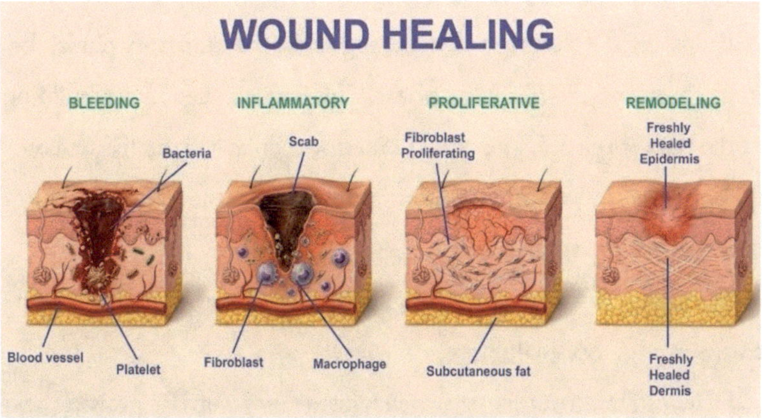


The first step in healing is inflammation, which is basically your body's "cleanup crew" getting to work. Right after you get hurt, your blood vessels tighten to stop the bleeding. Then, they open back up to let a rush of blood—and your immune system's "first responders"—into the wound. These special white blood cells act like a waste management team, clearing out dirt, bacteria, and dead skin. This cleaning stage is vital because a "dirty" wound can't heal right.

If it gets infected, the healing process takes much longer and is way more likely to leave a noticeable scar.

Think of macrophages as the "generals" of the healing process. Their job is to swallow up dirt and germs, but they also send out chemical signals to tell the rest of the body it's time to start rebuilding. This cleanup phase is a delicate balance.

You need enough inflammation to get the wound clean, but if the "cleanup crew" stays too long or works too hard, it can actually cause damage.

This overreaction is often what leads to thick, red, or bumpy scars like hypertrophic scars and keloids.

Following the cleanup and signalling of the inflammatory phase, the body enters the **proliferation phase**. This is where the actual rebuilding of the tissue begins. It's a period of intense cellular activity focused on filling the wound space and restoring the dermal structure. Several key events characterize this phase:

During the next phase of healing, your body focuses on rebuilding the tissue through two main steps:

First, it starts angiogenesis, which is just a fancy word for growing new blood vessels. These tiny pipes sprout to bring oxygen and nutrients to the injury. This extra blood flow is exactly why healing wounds look red and slightly bumpy.

Second, cells called fibroblasts move in to build a "patch." These cells produce collagen, the protein that gives your skin its strength. To close the gap quickly, the fibroblasts lay down the collagen in a messy, random pattern—kind of like a quick patch job on a road.

This initial collagen is also a weaker type (Type III) meant for speed, not strength.

Over time, your body replaces it with stronger collagen (Type I), but it never looks as neat or organized as your original, uninjured skin.

While the deeper layers are being patched with collagen, the surface of your skin also begins to repair itself through a process called epithelialization.

New skin cells (called keratinocytes) crawl from the edges of the wound toward the centre to create a fresh, thin top layer. This acts as a protective shield, sealing the wound off from the outside world and germs. In deeper cuts, this new skin grows right over the "filler" tissue that has already filled in the gap. Think of this "rebuilding phase" as a speedy construction project. Your body creates granulation tissue, which is a delicate, pink, lumpy layer made of new blood vessels and collagen.

This tissue acts as a temporary scaffold to fill the hole left by your injury. While it's necessary to close the wound, your body often overbuilds it. It piles on extra collagen just to make sure the seal is strong, which is exactly why scars can end up looking raised or bumpy instead of perfectly smooth like your original skin.

The final, and longest, phase of wound healing is **remodelling**, also known as maturation. This phase can begin as early as two to three weeks after injury and can continue for months, even up to two years or more. During remodelling, the wound tissue is reorganized, strengthened, and reshaped. It's a process of refinement and consolidation, where the initially fragile repair tissue matures into a more durable scar.

The most significant event during remodelling is the **collagen turnover and reorganization**. The abundant, disorganized collagen laid down during proliferation is gradually broken down and replaced with a stronger, more aligned network of Type I collagen.

This process is driven by specialized cells called myofibroblasts, which contract and pull the wound edges together, reducing the surface area of the scar. This contraction is essential for wound closure but can also contribute to tightness and restricted movement if the scar is located over a joint.

The tensile strength of the healing wound increases significantly during this phase, although it rarely reaches the full strength of uninjured skin (typically around 70-80%). The excessive vascularity also diminishes, causing the scar to fade from its initial bright red colour to a paler, more subdued hue. The scar tissue flattens and softens as the collagen fibres align and mature.

This remodelling phase is the "finishing touch" that determines what your scar will look like for years to come. Your body spends this time trying to find a perfect balance: it needs to break down the old, messy "patch" and replace it with stronger, neater collagen. If your body makes too much or doesn't tidy up well enough, the scar stays thick and bumpy. If it doesn't make enough or breaks it down too fast, the scar ends up thin and weak.

How your body handles this cleanup determines if the scar eventually fades and flattens or stays noticeable. The visual manifestation of these biological processes is what we perceive as a scar. It is, in essence, the body's attempt to create a functional repair rather than an exact replica of the original tissue. The inflammatory phase, with its vital cleanup and signalling, can sometimes overstay its welcome, leading to persistent redness and thickness. The proliferation phase, driven by a rush to close the wound, deposits a large volume of collagen in a disorganized manner, forming the initial raised and firm scar.

The remodelling phase then works to refine this structure, but the inherent difference in collagen organization and the overall cellular makeup means the repaired tissue will always differ from the original.

Understanding these phases—inflammation, proliferation, and remodelling—provides the crucial foundation for grasping why scars form. They are not aberrations but rather the natural, albeit imperfect, outcome of the body's healing processes. The characteristics of a scar – its colour, texture, thickness, and even its location and symptoms like itching or tightness – are all direct reflections of how efficiently and effectively these biological phases have unfolded. For example, a scar that remains red and raised for an extended period often indicates an ongoing or exaggerated inflammatory response or continued excessive collagen production during proliferation and early remodelling.

Conversely, an atrophic scar, one that appears indented, might suggest a deficit in collagen deposition or an aggressive inflammatory response that destroyed some of the underlying dermal structure.

The remarkable biological cascade of wound healing is a testament to the body's resilience and adaptive capabilities.

It is a multi-step, highly regulated process involving a complex interplay of cells, proteins, and signalling molecules.

From the initial inflammatory response that cleanses the wound and sets the stage, through the proliferative phase where new tissue is rapidly built with abundant collagen, to the prolonged remodelling phase where this tissue is refined and strengthened, each step is crucial. The resulting scar is a visible record of this intricate dance, a testament to the body's ability to repair itself, even if the repair is not a perfect restoration of the original.

By appreciating these fundamental biological underpinnings, we can move forward to understand the factors that influence scar appearance and explore the various methods available to optimize the healing process and improve the aesthetic and functional outcomes of scars. This foundational knowledge demystifies the scar and empowers us to approach its management with a deeper understanding of the body's own story of healing.

Think of collagen as the "steel rebar" inside a concrete building—it's the hidden support that gives your skin its strength, shape, and bounce. In healthy skin, these collagen fibres are neatly organized in parallel rows. This tidy setup lets your skin stretch and snap back into place without losing its form.

Most of this structure is made of Type I collagen (the strongest kind) and a bit of Type III collagen (which adds flexibility).

Together, they create a tough but stretchy framework that helps your skin handle movement and pressure while staying smooth and firm.

However, when the skin sustains an injury, this precise architectural blueprint is disrupted. The body's immediate response, as we've discussed, is to initiate a rapid repair process. Central to this repair is a surge in collagen production.

Fibroblasts, those industrious cellular architects, switch from their normal maintenance duties to a frenzied state of collagen synthesis. They begin churning out collagen in massive quantities, a biological imperative to quickly fill the void left by the injury and seal the breach in the skin's protective barrier. This initial wave of collagen deposition during the proliferation phase is characterized by a less organized, almost haphazard arrangement.

Instead of the neat, parallel bundles of healthy dermis, the collagen fibres are laid down in a more random, basket-weave pattern. This disorganized deposition is crucial for rapid wound closure, providing immediate structural support, but it fundamentally alters the tissue's properties.

Moreover, the type of collagen produced in the early stages of wound healing also differs. While Type I collagen is eventually favoured as the scar matures, the initial deposited collagen is often richer in Type III collagen. This type, while contributing to the overall bulk, is less organized and more extensible than mature Type I collagen, contributing to the initial softness and less defined structure of the developing scar. The sheer volume of collagen being deposited, coupled with its disorganized architecture, is the primary reason why scars are typically thicker and more raised than the surrounding healthy skin. The body, in its haste to repair, overbuilds, creating a patch rather than a seamless restoration.

To picture the difference, think of a perfectly built brick wall where every brick is straight and smooth. That represents your healthy, uninjured skin.

Now, imagine there's a hole in that wall and someone does an emergency repair by quickly piling in bricks however they fit. While the pile fills the hole and does the job, it looks messy and isn't as smooth or strong as the rest of the wall.

That "quick fix" is exactly how the collagen looks in a brand-new scar. The journey of collagen doesn't end with its initial deposition. The subsequent remodelling phase is dedicated to refining this hastily constructed matrix.

During this extended period, fibroblasts and specialized cells called myofibroblasts engage in a continuous process of collagen breakdown and synthesis. Think of it as a renovation project. The initial, disorganized scaffolding is gradually dismantled, and the remaining collagen fibres are realigned and strengthened. Myofibroblasts, with their contractile capabilities, play a significant role here, pulling the collagen fibres closer together, increasing the tensile strength of the scar tissue. This reorganization leads to a more parallel alignment of collagen fibres, albeit never achieving the perfect organization of uninjured skin.

The type of collagen also shifts during remodelling. There is a gradual replacement of Type III collagen with the stronger, more mature Type I collagen. This transition, along with the improved alignment, contributes to the scar's eventual flattening, softening, and paling. As the density of fibroblasts and blood vessels decreases, the scar loses its initial redness and becomes less prominent. However, the fundamental difference in the arrangement and composition of collagen fibres means that scar tissue will always possess a different quality than original dermal tissue. It will be less elastic, have a reduced ability to withstand stretching in certain directions, and may never regain the full strength of uninjured skin, typically reaching only 70-80% of its original tensile strength.

The quality and quantity of collagen produced and remodelled are directly influenced by various factors. Genetic predisposition plays a role, with some individuals inherently producing more robust or disorganized collagen. The depth and nature of the injury are also critical. A deep wound requiring significant tissue regeneration will naturally involve a more extensive collagen deposition than a superficial graze.

The inflammatory response, as discussed previously, also heavily influences collagen. A prolonged or excessive inflammatory phase can lead to continued fibroblast stimulation and overproduction of collagen, resulting in hypertrophic scars or keloids, where the scar tissue continues to grow beyond the original wound boundaries.

Conversely, an insufficient inflammatory response or a failure in fibroblast activity might lead to inadequate collagen deposition, resulting in atrophic scars. These scars appear indented because there simply isn't enough collagen to fill the defect and support the overlying epidermis. The body's attempt to create a strong repair, by depositing large amounts of collagen, can therefore paradoxically lead to a less aesthetically pleasing outcome if that collagen is not properly organized or if its production is unbalanced.

The visible characteristics of a scar are a direct consequence of this collagen story. The redness of a new scar is due to the increased vascularity that accompanies collagen production. The thickness and raised appearance are a result of the sheer volume of collagen deposited during proliferation. The texture, whether smooth or rough, is determined by the degree of organization and alignment of the collagen fibres.

The tightness and lack of pliability often associated with scars, particularly over joints, are due to the dense, less elastic network of collagen.

Understanding collagen's role is paramount because it is the primary target of many scar treatment modalities.

Treatments aim to influence collagen production, breakdown, or organization.

For instance, silicone sheeting and gels are thought to hydrate the scar tissue, potentially influencing fibroblast activity and collagen synthesis, leading to a softer, flatter scar. Laser therapies can target collagen by breaking down excessive deposits or stimulating remodelling. Microneedling creates micro-injuries that trigger the body's wound healing response, encouraging the production of new, more organized collagen. Surgical revision aims to physically rearrange or excise existing scar tissue, allowing the body to form a new scar with potentially improved collagen organization.

In essence, collagen is both the hero and the villain in your skin's healing story.

It is the essential "building material" that patches you up, but because your body is in such a rush to close a wound, it tends to overproduce collagen and pile it up in a messy way. This "rush job" is exactly what creates a visible scar.

The long remodelling process is just your body's way of trying to fix that messy first draft. It slowly tries to tidy up the pile and make the repair look and feel more like your original skin. By understanding how collagen moves from a "frantic patch" to a "neatly organized" structure, we can better choose treatments to help the process along.

The narrative of scar formation, as we've begun to uncover, is intricately woven into the biological tapestry of wound healing.

We've delved into the fundamental processes, focusing on the deposition and remodelling of collagen – the very scaffolding of our skin.

This journey of repair, however, is not a uniform one.

It is profoundly influenced by a confluence of intrinsic and extrinsic factors, each contributing to the unique character and appearance of the scar that ultimately graces our skin. To truly comprehend the story etched by a scar, we must acknowledge these modulating forces, understanding that the body's response to injury is a highly individualized phenomenon.

Among the most significant intrinsic determinants of scar appearance is our **genetics**. Our genetic makeup acts as a blueprint, dictating a multitude of cellular processes, including the way our bodies orchestrate wound repair and collagen synthesis. Some individuals are genetically predisposed to a more robust inflammatory response, which, while effective in combating infection, can also prolong the proliferation phase of healing. This prolonged phase means more fibroblasts are active for longer, churning out greater quantities of collagen. Moreover, genetic variations can influence the very type and quality of collagen produced, as well as the efficiency of the remodelling phase. For instance, certain gene polymorphisms have been associated with an increased likelihood of developing hypertrophic scars or keloids.

These are scars that grow beyond the boundaries of the original wound, a testament to an overzealous and dysregulated collagen production driven by genetic programming.

In essence, our genes can predispose us to either a more subtle, well-integrated repair or a more conspicuous, raised, and sometimes even actively growing scar.

This inherent variability means that two people sustaining identical injuries, under identical conditions, might experience vastly different healing outcomes purely based on their genetic inheritance.

The predisposition to form keloids, for example, is significantly more common in individuals of African, Asian, and Hispanic descent, highlighting a clear genetic component to this specific type of scar.

This isn't to say that everyone from these backgrounds will develop keloids, but rather that their genetic makeup confers a higher susceptibility compared to other populations.

Understanding this genetic influence is crucial because it helps set realistic expectations.

If there's a family history of prominent scarring, it's likely that an individual will also tend towards more noticeable scars, and treatments may need to be approached with this in mind, perhaps with a focus on early intervention and preventative strategies.

Closely intertwined with genetics, and often influencing the intensity of the genetic predisposition, is **age**.

The age of the individual at the time of injury plays a remarkable role in the trajectory of wound healing and, consequently, the resulting scar.

Younger skin, brimming with youthful vitality, typically possesses a more vigorous and accelerated healing response.

This heightened cellular activity, driven by a robust inflammatory cascade and a high rate of fibroblast proliferation, can lead to a more pronounced deposition of collagen in the initial stages.

While this ensures rapid wound closure and a strong initial repair, it also increases the likelihood of developing thicker, more raised scars, such as hypertrophic scars. The body of a child or adolescent is essentially geared for rapid growth and repair, and this translates into a more aggressive approach to wound healing.

Imagine a young, energetic construction crew tasked with repairing a damaged wall; they are likely to work quickly and perhaps a bit too enthusiastically, resulting in a substantial, albeit potentially uneven, patch. Conversely, as we age, our skin's capacity for rapid repair diminishes. The inflammatory response becomes less pronounced, fibroblast activity slows, and the overall healing process extends over a longer period. While this might suggest a reduced risk of hypertrophic scarring, older skin is more prone to developing atrophic scars. This is because the slower healing process and reduced collagen production may not be sufficient to fully fill the wound defect, leading to a sunken appearance as the surrounding skin loses volume over time. Furthermore, older skin is often thinner and less elastic due to decreased collagen and elastin production over years of exposure to environmental factors and intrinsic aging processes. This can make scars, even if not hypertrophic, appear more fragile and potentially more visible against the backdrop of thinning skin.

The hormonal changes associated with different life stages also contribute. For instance, the fluctuations in hormones during puberty can sometimes exacerbate scarring tendencies. Therefore, the age at which a wound occurs is not just a number; it's a biological marker that significantly shapes the healing narrative and the resulting scar.

A scar on a young child might be initially red and raised but could potentially soften and flatten more effectively over time as their body continues its remodelling processes. A similar scar on an older adult might remain flatter from the outset but could be more prone to developing a thinner, more noticeable appearance due to the surrounding skin's reduced resilience.

Beyond the intrinsic biological factors of genetics and age, the **location of the wound on the body** emerges as a critical extrinsic determinant of scar formation. The skin is not uniform across our entire anatomy; it varies in thickness, elasticity, and the underlying tension it experiences. Areas subjected to constant movement and stretching, such as over joints (elbows, knees), the chest, or the shoulders, are inherently more prone to developing prominent scars. These areas are under significant mechanical stress. When a wound heals in such a location, the forces of tension constantly pull at the healing tissue. This continuous traction can disrupt the delicate process of collagen remodelling. Instead of aligning in a neat, organized fashion, the collagen fibres are forced into a more chaotic, linear orientation, dictated by the direction of the pull. This leads to scars that are often wider, thicker, and more contracted than they might be in areas of lower tension. Think of trying to mend a tear in a fabric that is constantly being pulled taut – the mend will likely be strained and less smooth than if the fabric were relaxed. This is precisely what happens to healing skin under tension. The body's attempt to create a strong, stable repair in a high-tension zone often results in a scar that is itself under tension, leading to a contracted and sometimes functionally limiting outcome.

For example, a scar across a joint can restrict the range of motion, making it difficult to bend or straighten the limb.

The sternum, located on the anterior chest, is another area notorious for producing raised and thickened scars, particularly keloids. This is thought to be due to the constant stretching of the skin over the chest wall, combined with the skin's inherent predisposition to react robustly in this region.

Conversely, areas with less inherent tension and more laxity, such as the inner forearm or the abdomen (away from the linea alba), may heal with flatter, less noticeable scars, assuming other factors are equal. The thickness of the dermis itself also plays a role; areas with thicker skin, like the back, might involve a greater volume of collagen deposition during healing, potentially leading to more substantial scars. The vascularity of an area can also influence scar appearance. Areas with a richer blood supply might appear redder for longer. Therefore, when considering the potential outcome of a wound, the specific anatomical location is an indispensable piece of the puzzle. A small cut on the face might heal with a relatively inconspicuous scar due to lower tension and good blood supply, while a similar-sized injury on the back of the hand, constantly exposed to movement and potential friction, could develop into a more visible and potentially problematic scar. This understanding is crucial for managing expectations and for tailoring treatment strategies; scar revision techniques, for example, often aim to reposition scars into natural skin lines or areas of lower tension to improve their appearance and function.

It is vital to recognize that these factors—genetics, age, and location—do not operate in isolation.

They interact in complex ways, creating a unique landscape for each individual's healing journey. For instance, a genetically predisposed individual (prone to keloids) who sustains an injury in a high-tension area like the chest during their youth is at a significantly elevated risk of developing a severe, widespread keloid scar. Conversely, an older individual with a genetic predisposition for less robust healing might experience a shallower scar in a low-tension area.

The interplay between these elements underscores why no two scars are ever truly identical. Each scar tells a story, not just of the injury itself, but of the individual's unique biological context at the moment of healing. Acknowledging these inherent influences, while we cannot change them, empowers us. It allows for a more realistic assessment of potential scar outcomes and informs the selection of appropriate management and treatment strategies. It is the first step in understanding that while we might not control the initial hand fate has dealt us in terms of our genetic makeup, age, and where on our body an injury occurs, we can certainly learn to understand the story these factors contribute to our scar and make informed decisions about how to best support our skin's continued healing and recovery.

The intricate dance of healing, initiated by injury, is orchestrated by a sophisticated internal defence system: the immune system. Far from being a passive bystander, it is the proactive commander of the repair process, deploying its cellular legions to clear the battlefield, neutralize threats, and lay the groundwork for reconstruction. When the skin's integrity is breached, whether by a superficial scrape or a deep laceration, a cascade of immune events is immediately triggered.

This response is not a singular event but a dynamic, multi-phased operation, each stage crucial for successful wound resolution.

At the forefront of this defence are the neutrophils, a type of white blood cell that acts as the initial rapid-response force.

These phagocytic powerhouses are the first responders, migrating in large numbers to the injured site within minutes to hours.

Their primary mission is to engulf and digest cellular debris, foreign particles, and any invading microorganisms that may have entered through the compromised barrier.

This meticulous cleanup is essential not only to prevent infection but also to create a clear space for the subsequent repair processes to begin. Imagine them as the demolition crew, swiftly removing rubble and hazardous materials from a construction site. The presence of neutrophils is a hallmark of the early inflammatory phase, and their short lifespan means they are typically replaced by a different set of immune cells within a few days.

Right after the first responders (neutrophils) arrive, the macrophages take over. Think of them as the versatile managers of the healing process. They don't just clean up the remaining dirt and germs; they also act as conductors, sending out a "symphony" of chemical signals.

These signals do three big things: Call for builders: They recruit fibroblasts, the cells that make new collagen. Build new plumbing: They start angiogenesis, which is just growing new blood vessels to bring in oxygen and nutrients. Quiet the alarm: They tell the body to stop the inflammation once the area is safe and clean.

When these "manager" cells arrive, it's a sign that your body is moving from a defensive "emergency mode" into the actual rebuilding phase. This inflammatory phase, characterized by redness, swelling, heat, and pain, is a necessary and beneficial part of wound healing. It is the body's way of preparing the tissue for repair. However, like any powerful biological process, the immune response must be carefully regulated.

The balance of this inflammatory cascade is paramount.

If the inflammatory response is too weak or is suppressed, the wound may struggle to clear debris, fight off infection, and initiate repair effectively, leading to delayed healing, chronic wounds, or increased susceptibility to infection.

If the "cleanup crew" (inflammation) stays at the wound site for too long, it can cause problems for your scar.

When these immune cells don't leave, they keep shouting at the "builder" cells (fibroblasts) to keep making collagen. This constant "on" switch leads to two types of thick, bumpy scars:

Hypertrophic scars: These stay within the edges of the original cut. They are thick and raised, but they often get better or flatter as time goes on.

Keloids: These are more aggressive. They don't just stay in the wound; they spread into the healthy skin around it and almost never go away on their own.

Basically, the lingering inflammation keeps telling your body to "keep building," resulting in a pile-up of scar tissue that shouldn't be there. The role of specific inflammatory cells, such as mast cells and cytokines, is also being increasingly understood in the context of scar formation.

Mast cells are the same cells that cause allergic reactions, and they wake up whenever you get an injury.

They release histamine (the stuff that makes you itchy) and other powerful chemicals that act like "loudspeakers" for your immune system. These chemicals tell your body to keep the inflammation going and keep your "builder" cells (fibroblasts) working overtime.

If these cells stay active for too long, they create a cycle where your body thinks it needs to keep making collagen forever.

This constant "build" signal is a huge reason why thick, bumpy hypertrophic scars and keloids form.

This understanding of the immune system's crucial role in wound healing and scar formation opens avenues for therapeutic interventions. Modulating the inflammatory response can be a key strategy in managing scar appearance. For instance, early interventions aimed at dampening excessive inflammation, such as the topical or intralesional application of corticosteroids, are often employed to reduce the redness, thickness, and itching associated with hypertrophic scars and keloids. These agents work by inhibiting the inflammatory cascade and reducing fibroblast proliferation.

Similarly, other treatments that target inflammatory pathways, such as silicone sheeting or pressure therapy, are believed to work, in part, by reducing local inflammation and altering the signalling environment within the healing wound.

The immune system's involvement in scar formation highlights the body's remarkable, yet sometimes imperfect, capacity for self-repair.

The process is a delicate balancing act. When functioning optimally, it leads to seamless closure and minimal residual evidence of injury.

However, when this intricate immune orchestration falters, or when the inflammatory signals become too persistent, the result can be scars that are not only aesthetically concerning but can also lead to functional limitations and chronic discomfort. Recognizing the immune system as a central player in this narrative provides a deeper appreciation for the complex biological processes that govern how our skin heals and why some scars become prominent features, while others fade into near invisibility.

It underscores that the story of a scar is, in many ways, the story of the body's immune defence and repair mechanisms at work, a testament to our inherent resilience and the intricate biological machinery that seeks to restore our integrity.

The journey from a wound to a scar is not an instantaneous event but rather a dynamic and often lengthy process of biological transformation. Following the initial stages of inflammation and repair, where the body diligently works to close the breach in the skin's protective barrier, the newly formed tissue begins a period of maturation. This maturation phase is where the visible characteristics of the scar begin to refine, evolve, and ultimately stabilize. Understanding this natural timeline is crucial for setting realistic expectations and appreciating the body's inherent capacity for healing. It is a story of gradual change, marked by shifts in colour, texture, and sensitivity, a visible testament to the complex cellular ballet that occurred beneath the surface.

In the immediate aftermath of wound closure, the nascent scar is typically characterized by its vibrant, often angry, red hue. This redness is a direct consequence of the intense vascularization that occurred during the proliferative phase of healing. New blood vessels, essential for delivering oxygen and nutrients to the rebuilding tissue, proliferate rapidly to support the fibroblast activity. While these vessels are vital for healing, their abundance in the immature scar lends it a prominent, raised, and often tender appearance. The skin in this area may feel warm to the touch, further indicating the heightened metabolic activity and increased blood flow. This early phase can be somewhat alarming, as the scar often appears much more noticeable and discoloured than one might hope for.

However, it is a critical, albeit temporary, stage in the scar's evolution. The skin's natural response to injury involves a surge of blood supply to facilitate the delivery of crucial healing components, and this influx is clearly visible in the scar's initial coloration.

Over the ensuing weeks and months, this initial redness begins to gradually subside.

As the wound matures and the demand for nutrients and oxygen lessens, the excess blood vessels in the scar tissue start to regress.

This reduction in vascularity is directly responsible for the scar lightening in colour, transitioning from the initial bright red towards a more muted pink, and eventually, to a pale, off-white, or even slightly darker tone than the surrounding skin.

This lightening process is not uniform and can vary significantly depending on individual skin types and the depth of the original injury.

For individuals with lighter skin tones, the scar may become noticeably lighter than their natural complexion, sometimes appearing almost translucent. Conversely, in those with darker skin, the scar might retain more pigment, appearing pink, brown, or even hyperpigmented, meaning it is darker than the surrounding skin. This variation in pigment is influenced by the activity of melanocytes, the cells responsible for producing melanin, the pigment that gives skin its colour. In some instances, particularly with deeper wounds or in individuals prone to

hyperpigmentation, the scar may remain noticeably darker than the surrounding skin for an extended period, or even permanently. This darkening is often a result of inflammatory triggers stimulating melanocyte activity.

At the same time the texture of the scar undergoes a significant transformation. The initial raised and often firm quality of the immature scar begins to soften and flatten. The overabundance of collagen, initially laid down in a somewhat disorganized fashion to quickly bridge the wound, starts to remodel. This remodelling process, guided by fibroblasts and influenced by mechanical forces, realigns the collagen fibres, making them more parallel and organized. As this reorganization progresses, the scar tissue becomes less dense and more pliable. The once prominent, raised appearance gradually yields to a flatter, smoother surface.

This flattening can take many months, sometimes even a year or more, to become fully apparent.

It is a gradual metamorphosis, where the initial bulky deposit of repair tissue is refined into a more integrated and less conspicuous part of the skin. The feeling of tightness and hardness associated with a new scar typically diminishes as this collagen remodelling continues, contributing to a more comfortable and less noticeable final scar.

Sensitivity is another characteristic that evolves over time. Newly formed scars are often hypersensitive, prone to itching, burning, and pain upon touch. This heightened sensitivity is a result of the numerous nerve endings that are present in the immature scar tissue. As the scar matures, these nerve endings either recede or become less reactive, and the scar tissue itself becomes less inflamed and more integrated with the surrounding skin. The itching, a common and often frustrating symptom of healing wounds and scars, typically subsides as the inflammatory response diminishes and the epidermal barrier is fully restored.

While some residual sensitivity might persist in certain areas or with specific stimuli, the acute tenderness and itching usually diminish considerably within the first year of the scar's formation. This gradual reduction in sensitivity is a welcome sign of the scar's ongoing maturation and integration into the surrounding tissues.

The timeline for these changes is highly variable and influenced by a multitude of factors, including the individual's age, genetics, skin type, the location and depth of the wound, and the quality of the initial wound care. Generally, the most rapid changes in colour and texture occur within the first three to six months. During this period, the scar will noticeably flatten, lighten, and soften.

However, the maturation process continues long after this initial period. Significant improvements in appearance can still be observed up to 18 to 24 months post-injury. It is important for individuals to understand that a scar is a dynamic entity, constantly undergoing subtle changes for up to two years or even longer. This prolonged maturation period means that even scars that appear unfavourable in the early stages have a good chance of improving considerably over time with the body's natural healing processes.

It is also worth noting that scars rarely disappear completely. The goal of scar maturation is not erasure but rather assimilation. A mature scar typically appears as a fine line, less noticeable in colour and texture compared to its initial state. It should blend more harmoniously with the surrounding skin, becoming less of a distinct feature and more of an integrated part of the skin's landscape. The final appearance can range from a barely perceptible silvery line to a slightly discoloured or textured area, depending on the factors mentioned earlier.

Patience is a key virtue when observing scar evolution. Rushing to judgment or undertaking aggressive interventions too early can sometimes be counterproductive. Allowing the body its natural course of healing and maturation is often the most effective strategy for achieving the best possible aesthetic outcome. This understanding of the natural trajectory of scar development serves as a foundational perspective, providing a clear picture of what to anticipate before exploring various methods to further refine or manage the scar's appearance. The body's innate ability to heal and remodel is a remarkable process, and observing this transition from a raw wound to a mature scar offers a profound insight into our biological resilience.

# CHAPTER THREE

## Topical Treatments and Home Care: First Lines of Defence

The realm of non-invasive scar management has long sought a universally effective, accessible, and patient-friendly solution. For decades, silicone-based products have emerged as a leading contender, often hailed as the "gold standard" in topical scar treatment.

Their widespread availability, ease of use, and compelling anecdotal and clinical evidence have solidified their position in the dermatologist's and plastic surgeon's armamentarium.

But what exactly is it about silicone that renders it so effective?

And how can patients best leverage these products for optimal results?

At its core, the proposed efficacy of silicone in scar management hinges on a multifaceted approach, primarily involving the creation of a favourable microenvironment for healing and the modulation of the underlying cellular processes that contribute to scar formation.

One of the most widely accepted mechanisms is the **hydration of the stratum corneum**, the outermost layer of the epidermis.

When silicone is applied, particularly in the form of sheeting, it forms a semi-occlusive barrier.

This barrier effectively reduces trans epidermal water loss (TEWL), preventing excessive dehydration of the scar tissue.

By maintaining optimal hydration, the stratum corneum remains supple and pliable, which is crucial for preventing the formation of dry, brittle scar tissue that can lead to itching and irritation. This hydrated state also supports the natural desquamation process, the shedding of dead skin cells, which can contribute to a smoother scar surface. Think of it as keeping a wound moist to promote better healing – silicone sheeting achieves a similar effect on the surface of a healing scar, preventing it from becoming overly dry and constricted. This prolonged hydration can also influence the underlying dermal layers by altering the extracellular matrix.

Beyond surface-level hydration, silicone is believed to exert more profound biochemical effects on the scar tissue itself. Research suggests that silicone plays a role in **regulating fibroblast growth factors**. Fibroblasts are the primary cells responsible for producing collagen, the structural protein that forms scar tissue. In the process of scar formation, fibroblasts can become overactive, leading to the excessive deposition of collagen, which results in raised and thickened scars like hypertrophic scars and keloids. Silicone's interaction with these growth factors, such as transforming growth factor-beta (TGF- ), is thought to downregulate fibroblast proliferation and collagen synthesis. By tempering the fibroblasts' exuberance, silicone helps to prevent the overproduction of collagen that characterizes problematic scarring. This modulation helps to guide the scar towards a more organized and less exuberant matrix, promoting a flatter and softer outcome.

Furthermore, silicone is implicated in **preventing collagen cross-linking**. Collagen molecules are naturally cross-linked to provide strength and structure to tissues.

However, in scar tissue, this cross-linking process can become dysregulated, leading to stiff, contracted collagen bundles. This aberrant cross-linking contributes to the raised, firm, and sometimes contracted appearance of hypertrophic scars and keloids.

Silicone is thought to interfere with the enzymes responsible for this excessive cross-linking, such as lysyl oxidase.

By inhibiting this process, silicone helps to break down the rigid collagen matrix and promote the formation of a more organized, flexible, and less fibrotic scar tissue.

This reduction in cross-linking is directly responsible for the softening and flattening effect observed in treated scars.

The concept of silicone as a "gold standard" is supported by its versatility in application. The most recognizable form is **silicone sheeting**. These are thin, flexible, and adhesive sheets made from medical-grade silicone. They are designed to be cut to size and applied directly to the scar.

The sheeting offers continuous contact with the scar tissue, ensuring consistent hydration and modulation of cellular activity.

They are typically worn for extended periods, often 12-24 hours a day, and can be reused for several days or weeks, depending on the product and adherence to cleaning instructions.

The adherence of the sheets can vary, and some users may benefit from additional medical tape to secure them, especially in areas with a lot of movement.

The sheets are generally well-tolerated, but occasional mild redness or itching can occur, usually due to the adhesive or trapped moisture.

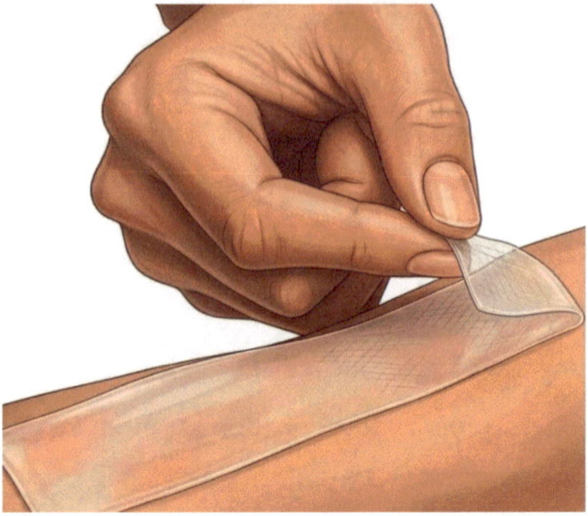

Another prevalent form is **silicone gel**. These are typically clear, fast-drying formulations that can be applied directly to the scar surface. Gels offer a more convenient option for individuals who find sheeting cumbersome or uncomfortable, especially on curved or mobile areas of the body. They are applied in a thin layer, forming a breathable, waterproof barrier that provides similar benefits to the sheeting, albeit with potentially less sustained occlusion. Gels are typically applied multiple times a day, often two to three times, depending on the product's instructions. The drying time is usually rapid, allowing for immediate dressing or clothing application. Silicone gels are particularly well-suited for facial scars, areas with hair, or regions where traditional sheeting might be difficult to apply or maintain. The texture of the gel is often smooth and non-greasy, making it a pleasant option for daily use.

For even greater convenience and discretion, **silicone sprays** have also gained popularity. These aerosolized formulations allow for a light, even coating of silicone over the scar. They are ideal for covering larger areas or for individuals who prefer a hands-free application.

Like gels, sprays create a breathable barrier and are applied multiple times a day.

The fine mist ensures even distribution without the need for rubbing, which can be beneficial for sensitive scar tissue. However, some sprays may be less occlusive than sheeting or gels, potentially offering a slightly different level of efficacy.

The ease of application makes them a strong contender for maintaining consistent treatment, especially for patients who struggle with the routine of applying gels or sheeting.

Regardless of the form chosen, consistent and prolonged application is paramount for achieving optimal results. The **recommended usage** for silicone sheeting and gels generally involves continuous wear for the sheets and multiple daily applications for gels and sprays, often for a minimum of 8-12 weeks, and sometimes up to six months or even longer, particularly for more mature or severe scars.

The duration of treatment often depends on the age and nature of the scar. Newer scars that are still in the active healing phase tend to respond more favorably and more rapidly to silicone therapy. However, even older, established scars can benefit from long-term treatment, as silicone can help to soften and flatten them over time.

Adherence is key; skipping applications or failing to wear the sheets for the recommended duration can significantly compromise the outcome. Patient education regarding the importance of consistency cannot be overstated.

The **evidence supporting the efficacy** of silicone-based treatments, particularly for hypertrophic and keloid scars, is substantial and continues to grow.

Numerous clinical studies, systematic reviews, and meta-analyses have demonstrated that silicone therapy is an effective first-line treatment for improving scar appearance, reducing scar elevation, alleviating scar-related symptoms such as itching and pain, and improving scar pliability. For instance, studies comparing silicone sheeting to no treatment or placebo treatments have consistently shown significant improvements in scar volume, height, and overall cosmetic outcome.

The American Academy of Dermatology and the European Wound Management Association have both recommended silicone gel sheeting as a primary treatment option for scars. While the exact percentage of improvement can vary widely depending on individual factors, scar type, and treatment duration, patients often report noticeable positive changes in their scars, leading to increased confidence and improved quality of life. The mechanisms of action, as discussed earlier, provide a strong biological rationale for this observed clinical benefit.

Despite its widespread acceptance and proven efficacy, adherence to silicone therapy can sometimes be a challenge for patients. **Practical tips for adherence and managing potential skin irritation** can significantly enhance the treatment experience.

For silicone sheeting, ensuring the skin is clean and dry before application is crucial for optimal adhesion. If the edges begin to lift, a small piece of medical tape can be used to secure them.

For individuals with sensitive skin or adhesive allergies, hypoallergenic tapes can be a helpful alternative.

Regular cleaning of the reusable sheets, as per the manufacturer's instructions (usually with mild soap and water), is essential to maintain their stickiness and prevent bacterial buildup.

If irritation occurs, such as redness, itching, or a rash, it is important to discontinue use and consult with a healthcare professional. Sometimes, the irritation is not from the silicone itself but from the adhesive or trapped moisture. Taking breaks from application, ensuring thorough cleaning, or switching to a different silicone formulation (e.g., from sheeting to gel) can resolve these issues.

When using silicone gels or sprays, applying a thin, even layer is more effective than a thick coating.

Allowing the product to dry completely before covering it with clothing or applying makeup is also important. For individuals prone to skin sensitivity, patch testing a small area of unaffected skin before applying to the scar can help identify potential reactions. Educating patients about the expected timeline for results is also vital; significant improvement may take several weeks to months, and patience is key. Some individuals may benefit from combining silicone therapy with other treatments, such as pressure therapy or massage, under the guidance of their physician.

Ultimately, the "gold standard" status of silicone in scar management is well-earned, stemming from its robust scientific backing, diverse product forms, ease of use, and remarkable ability to transform the appearance and feel of scars, offering a tangible path towards improved skin aesthetics and patient satisfaction.

The journey towards optimal scar healing and improved skin texture is deeply intertwined with the fundamental principle of hydration. While advanced topical treatments and procedures play significant roles, the consistent and judicious use of moisturizers and emollients forms a crucial, yet often understated, cornerstone of effective scar care.

These formulations work in concert with the skin's natural processes, providing a supportive environment that facilitates scar maturation and enhances overall skin quality. Far from being a mere cosmetic indulgence, proper moisturizing is an active strategy in managing the healing process, particularly during those critical early stages when the skin barrier is compromised and vulnerable.

At its core, the benefit of moisturizers and emollients lies in their ability to combat dryness and promote a more supple, pliable scar. Scar tissue, by its very nature, is often different from the surrounding healthy skin. It can be denser, have a different collagen structure, and may even possess a reduced capacity to retain moisture. This can lead to a scar that feels tight, itchy, and looks dull or uneven.

Emollients, in particular, are designed to smooth and soften the skin's surface. They work by filling in the microscopic gaps between skin cells, creating a smoother texture and reducing the roughness often associated with scar tissue. This physical smoothing effect can immediately make a scar feel more comfortable and appear less prominent.

Beyond surface smoothing, a key mechanism by which moisturizers contribute to scar healing is through the **maintenance of skin barrier function**. The stratum corneum, the outermost layer of the epidermis, acts as a critical protective shield.

It prevents excessive water loss from the body (trans epidermal water loss, or TEWL) and shields the underlying tissues from environmental aggressors. In areas of scar formation, this barrier can be disrupted. Moisturizers, especially those rich in humectants, draw water from deeper layers of the skin and the environment to hydrate the stratum corneum.

This increased hydration helps to reinforce the skin's natural barrier, making it more resilient and better equipped to heal. Think of it as providing essential building materials and optimal working conditions for the skin's repair crew. A well-hydrated barrier is less prone to irritation, inflammation, and the subsequent exacerbation of scar appearance.

The role of **emollients** in this process is equally vital. Unlike humectants, which draw moisture, emollients form a physical layer on the skin's surface. This layer acts as a protective occlusive or semi-occlusive barrier, significantly reducing TEWL. By trapping moisture within the skin, emollients prevent dehydration, which is a primary driver of dryness, flaking, and the uncomfortable tightness often experienced with healing scars. This sustained hydration allows the skin cells to function more effectively, promoting better cell turnover and facilitating the natural remodelling of collagen that occurs during scar maturation. The pliability that emollients impart is crucial; stiff, dry scar tissue is more likely to restrict movement and can contribute to a less favourable cosmetic outcome. By keeping the scar tissue soft and flexible, emollients help it integrate more seamlessly with the surrounding skin.

When selecting moisturizers and emollients for scar care, paying attention to key ingredients can significantly enhance their effectiveness. **Hyaluronic acid** is a potent humectant, renowned for its exceptional ability to attract and retain water. It can hold up to 1,000 times its weight in water, making it a powerful tool for deeply hydrating scar tissue. Its presence in topical formulations helps to plump the skin, reduce the appearance of fine lines often associated with dryness, and create a smoother surface.

Another class of ingredients that are foundational to skin barrier health are **ceramides**. These are lipids, or fats, that are naturally found in the skin and are essential components of the skin's barrier structure. They act like the mortar between the skin cells (the bricks), helping to hold them together and prevent water loss. In damaged or scarred skin, ceramide levels can be depleted. Replenishing them through topical application can significantly help to restore the skin's barrier function, improve hydration, and reduce sensitivity. Products containing ceramides are particularly beneficial for scars that feel compromised or are prone to irritation.

**Natural oils and butters** also play a significant role as emollients and occlusives, offering a rich source of nourishing fatty acids and vitamins. For instance, shea butter and cocoa butter are excellent sources of emollients that provide deep moisturization and help to soften and condition the skin. Jojoba oil, which closely mimics the skin's natural sebum, is well-tolerated and can help to balance oil production while providing hydration. Rosehip oil is another popular choice, rich in essential fatty acids and antioxidants, believed to support skin regeneration and improve scar appearance.

While these natural ingredients can be very effective, it's important to note that some individuals may have sensitivities or allergies to specific oils, so patch testing is always advisable.

The **importance of consistent application**, especially during the early stages of wound healing and scar formation, cannot be overstated. As soon as a wound has closed and is no longer open and weeping, initiating a regular moisturizing regimen is key.

During this period, the skin is actively rebuilding its barrier, and providing it with a consistent supply of hydration and emollient support can profoundly influence the final scar outcome. Applying moisturizers two to three times a day, or whenever the skin feels dry or tight, helps to prevent the scar from becoming hardened or excessively raised. This consistent hydration not only improves comfort by alleviating itching and tightness but also supports the delicate cellular processes involved in collagen remodelling. Think of it as a continuous nurturing process that guides the scar towards a more favourable maturation.

While moisturizers and emollients are not typically considered a primary treatment for significant scarring, such as established hypertrophic scars or keloids, their role in enhancing the skin's overall health and contributing to a smoother scar appearance is undeniable. They act as an adjunct therapy, working synergistically with other scar management techniques. By improving the skin's barrier function, moisturizers can help prevent secondary issues like infection or further inflammation that could negatively impact scar healing. Furthermore, by improving the texture and

suppleness of the scar, they can significantly enhance the patient's comfort and self-perception. A scar that feels softer and looks less dry is often perceived as less bothersome.

For individuals with **different skin types**, the choice of moisturizer might vary. Those with oily or acne-prone skin might prefer lighter, non-comedogenic formulations. Gel-based moisturizers or lotions containing hyaluronic acid and niacinamide can provide hydration without feeling heavy or clogging pores.

For individuals with dry or sensitive skin, richer creams and ointments containing ceramides, shea butter, or colloidal oatmeal are often more beneficial. These thicker formulations provide a more robust occlusive barrier, offering extended hydration and protection.

It's always prudent to select products that are fragrance-free and hypoallergenic, especially when applying to sensitive healing skin. Reading ingredient lists and understanding the specific needs of your skin can guide you towards the most effective product.

In essence, incorporating moisturizers and emollients into a scar care routine is an accessible, cost-effective, and essential step towards achieving the best possible outcome. They are the unsung heroes of scar management, working diligently to support the skin's natural healing cascade. By understanding the mechanisms by which they work and choosing products with beneficial ingredients, patients can harness the power of hydration to soften scar tissue, improve skin texture, and foster a smoother, more comfortable, and aesthetically pleasing scar. This commitment to consistent, supportive care, even in its simplest form, lays a vital foundation for the skin's journey towards recovery and resilience.

The quest for a smoother, less noticeable scar often leads individuals to the aisles of pharmacies and online retailers, where a vast array of topical creams and ointments are marketed for scar reduction. These products range from readily available over-the-counter (OTC) options to prescription-strength formulations, each promising to diminish the appearance of scars, improve texture, and restore skin's natural beauty. However, navigating this crowded market can be a daunting task, with claims often outpacing scientific evidence.

This subsection aims to critically examine the efficacy of these commonly found scar treatments, dissecting their active ingredients and evaluating the scientific backing behind their purported benefits. It is crucial to approach these products with a discerning eye, understanding that while some may offer modest improvements, they are generally not a panacea for significant scarring and should be viewed within the broader context of scar management.

One of the most ubiquitous ingredients found in many OTC scar creams is **onion extract**, often derived from *Allium cepa*. This natural extract has been a staple in some scar treatment formulations for decades, and its proponents suggest it possesses anti-inflammatory, antioxidant, and collagen-inhibiting properties. The theory behind its use is that it may help to soften scar tissue, reduce redness, and prevent the overproduction of collagen that leads to raised scars. Some early studies and anecdotal reports have indicated a potential benefit, particularly in improving scar pliability and reducing erythema. However, the scientific evidence supporting onion extract's efficacy is, at best, mixed and often lacks the robust, large-scale, placebo-controlled trials necessary to establish definitive proof. Many studies suffer from methodological limitations, such as small sample sizes, lack of standardized formulations, and subjective outcome measures. Furthermore, the concentration of onion extract can vary significantly between products, making it difficult to generalize results. While not typically associated with significant side effects, some individuals may experience mild skin irritation or allergic reactions. It is important to temper expectations; onion extract is unlikely to dramatically alter the appearance of mature or severe scars and may offer only subtle improvements for newer scars.

Another ingredient frequently touted for its scar-healing properties is **Vitamin E**. This fat-soluble antioxidant is a popular choice due to its perceived benefits in skin repair and protection. It is believed to play a role in reducing inflammation, promoting cell regeneration, and protecting against oxidative damage, all of which are relevant to wound healing.

However, despite its widespread use and intuitive appeal, the scientific literature on topical Vitamin E for scar treatment is largely disappointing. Several well-designed studies have failed to demonstrate any significant benefit in scar appearance compared to placebo or petrolatum alone.

In fact, some research has even suggested that topical Vitamin E may exacerbate scarring in certain individuals, leading to contact dermatitis or increased redness. The reason for this discrepancy between belief and evidence is not fully understood, but it's possible that the molecule's large size and lipid-soluble nature limit its penetration into deeper layers of the skin where scar remodelling primarily occurs. Additionally, the mechanism of action might be more relevant to systemic health rather than direct topical application for scar modulation. While Vitamin E is an essential nutrient and safe to use topically in many contexts, its efficacy for scar reduction remains questionable based on current scientific consensus.

**Heparin** and its derivatives are sometimes incorporated into scar treatment formulations, particularly those aimed at managing hypertrophic scars and keloids.

Heparin is a naturally occurring anticoagulant that also possesses anti-inflammatory and anti-proliferative properties.

In the context of scar management, it is thought to inhibit fibroblast proliferation and collagen synthesis, thereby potentially reducing scar thickness and improving its appearance. Some studies, particularly those conducted in certain regions, have suggested that topical heparin, often in combination with other agents like allantoin and onion extract (forming a combination often found in products like Mederma or Contractubex), may offer some benefit in softening scars and reducing inflammation. However, the quality of evidence supporting these claims can vary, and the concentration and vehicle in which heparin is delivered are critical factors. Similar to onion extract, the overall impact is generally considered to be mild, and it is unlikely to produce dramatic results on its own. The absorption of topical heparin into scar tissue is a key determinant of its effectiveness, and this can be influenced by the integrity of the skin barrier and the formulation itself.

**Allantoin**, a compound found in comfrey root and also synthesized chemically, is another ingredient commonly found in scar creams. It is prized for its soothing, moisturizing, and keratolytic properties. Allantoin is believed to promote cell proliferation and tissue regeneration, aid in the shedding of dead skin cells, and help to soften the skin, making it feel smoother. Its anti-inflammatory properties can also contribute to reducing redness and irritation associated with healing scars. Allantoin is generally well-tolerated and is often included in formulations as a complementary ingredient to enhance comfort and texture.

While it can contribute to improving the overall feel and hydration of the scar area, it is typically not considered a potent scar-reducing agent on its own.

Its primary role is often to support the skin's natural healing processes and improve superficial skin quality rather than to significantly alter the underlying collagen structure of a mature scar.

Beyond these commonly cited ingredients, many scar creams incorporate a proprietary blend of **silicones**, **moisturizers** (like petrolatum, mineral oil, glycerin), **antioxidants**, and other **botanicals**. Silicone-based products, in particular, have garnered significant attention and are often considered a gold standard among topical scar treatments.

While this subsection focuses on creams and ointments with specific active ingredients, it's worth noting that silicone sheeting and gels are frequently recommended by dermatologists and plastic surgeons.

Their mechanism of action is thought to involve hydration, occlusion, and a reduction in fibroblast activity, leading to softer, flatter scars. However, some silicone-based creams may contain lower concentrations of silicone compared to dedicated silicone gels or sheets, thus potentially offering less potent results.

When evaluating OTC scar creams and ointments, it is paramount to distinguish between compelling marketing claims and scientifically validated efficacy. Many products are formulated with a cocktail of ingredients, making it challenging to isolate the effect of any single component.

Furthermore, the "placebo effect" can play a significant role; the belief that a product is working can lead to subjective improvements in how a patient perceives their scar. This is not to dismiss the potential benefits of some formulations, but rather to advocate for realistic expectations.

For newer scars, or those with mild redness and superficial texture changes, a well-formulated cream containing humectants, emollients, and perhaps mild anti-inflammatory agents might offer some degree of improvement by supporting the skin's natural healing process and improving hydration. However, for more established, significant scarring such as deep indentations, wide atrophic scars, or raised hypertrophic and keloid scars, topical creams and ointments are generally insufficient as a standalone treatment.

The limitations of these over-the-counter products often lie in their penetration capabilities and the concentration of active ingredients. Scar tissue, particularly mature scar tissue, has a dense collagen matrix and altered vascularity, which can impede the penetration of topical agents. To achieve significant remodelling of scar collagen, more potent interventions are typically required. This is where prescription-strength formulations, professional treatments, and medical-grade devices come into play.

When choosing a scar cream or ointment, several factors should be considered. Firstly, look for products with a transparent ingredient list. Be wary of vague claims and "proprietary blends" that obscure the actual composition. Secondly, consider the type and age of your scar. Newer scars, especially those with inflammation and redness, might respond better to ingredients with anti-inflammatory and antioxidant properties. Older, more established scars may require treatments that can influence collagen remodelling more directly, which topical creams often struggle to achieve. Thirdly, consult with a dermatologist or plastic surgeon. They can assess your scar type and recommend treatments that are evidence-based and tailored to your specific needs.

They can also advise on the realistic outcomes achievable with topical agents versus other modalities.

It is also important to acknowledge that some ingredients, while natural, can cause irritation. Always perform a patch test on a small, inconspicuous area of skin before applying any new product to a scar, especially if your skin is sensitive. Fragrance-free and hypoallergenic formulations are generally preferred for scar care to minimize the risk of adverse reactions.

In summary, the landscape of over-the-counter and prescription scar creams and ointments is a complex one, characterized by a blend of traditional remedies, modern formulations, and significant marketing efforts. While ingredients like onion extract, vitamin E, heparin, and allantoin are frequently found in these products, the scientific evidence supporting their efficacy in significantly reducing scars is often limited, mixed, or inconclusive. Vitamin E, in particular, has shown little to no benefit in rigorous studies. Onion extract and heparin may offer mild improvements for some scars, especially in combination therapies, but are not miracle cures. Allantoin primarily offers soothing and moisturizing benefits. Ultimately, these topical treatments are best viewed as adjuncts to scar management, capable of providing some degree of superficial improvement, enhancing comfort, and supporting the skin's natural healing processes, particularly for newer or less severe scars. For more substantial scarring, a comprehensive approach involving medical-grade treatments and professional guidance remains the most effective strategy. The key is to maintain realistic expectations and prioritize evidence-based approaches when seeking to improve the appearance of scars.

Sun protection stands as a cornerstone of scar management, an often-underestimated yet critically important step in preventing long-term discoloration. As your skin heals and the scar tissue matures, it remains uniquely vulnerable to the damaging effects of ultraviolet (UV) radiation from the sun. Understanding this vulnerability is the first step toward effective prevention. Unlike the surrounding healthy skin, which contains a more robust and evenly distributed melanin pigment, scar tissue often lacks sufficient pigment or has an altered distribution of melanocytes. Melanin is the pigment responsible for skin's colour and acts as a natural defence against UV damage. When exposed to the sun, UV rays stimulate melanocytes to produce more melanin. In healthy skin, this leads to a tan. However, in scar tissue, this process can go awry.

The primary concern with sun exposure on scars is the risk of **hyperpigmentation**, commonly known as darkening. When UV rays penetrate the scar tissue, they can trigger an overproduction of melanin in the area. This is because the scar tissue, being newly formed or still in the process of remodelling, is more sensitive to external stimuli. The inflammatory response triggered by UV exposure can further exacerbate this pigment production. This leads to the scar becoming noticeably darker than the surrounding skin, often a reddish-brown or greyish-brown hue. This darkening can be persistent and, in some cases, may become permanent, making the scar even more conspicuous. This phenomenon is particularly prevalent in individuals with darker skin tones, as their melanocytes are already more active and responsive to stimuli. The contrast between a darkened scar and lighter surrounding skin can be a significant source of distress for many individuals seeking to minimize the visibility of their scars.

The altered vascularity within scar tissue can also contribute to a reddish or purplish hue, which can be further intensified by sun exposure.

Conversely, sun exposure can also lead to **hypopigmentation**, or lightening, of scars, though this is less common. In some instances, intense UV exposure or prolonged sun damage can actually damage the melanocytes within the scar tissue, leading to a reduction in melanin production. This results in the scar appearing lighter than the surrounding skin, creating a pale, whitish, or even chalky appearance. This type of discoloration is often more challenging to treat and can be more noticeable in individuals with darker skin tones, where the contrast with the lighter scar is more pronounced. Both hyperpigmentation and hypopigmentation represent a deviation from the scar's natural healing progression and can significantly impact its aesthetic outcome. The key takeaway is that unprotected sun exposure disrupts the delicate process of scar maturation and can lead to irreversible colour changes.

The timeline for this vulnerability is also important to consider. New scars, those that are still pink, red, or purplish, are the most susceptible to sun-induced darkening. This period typically lasts from a few months to a year or even longer after the initial injury or surgery, as the scar tissue continues to remodel and strengthen. During this active phase, the scar is essentially "open" to external influences, and UV radiation can wreak havoc on its developing pigmentary characteristics. Even after a scar has faded to a paler colour, it can still be prone to darkening with sun exposure. Therefore, a proactive and consistent approach to sun protection is not a short-term fix but a long-term commitment to achieving the best possible aesthetic outcome for your scar.

Given this heightened susceptibility, implementing rigorous sun protection strategies is not merely a recommendation; it is a necessity for anyone aiming to minimize scar discoloration. The most effective defence begins with **broad-spectrum sunscreen**. This means choosing a sunscreen that protects against both UVA and UVB rays. UVB rays are primarily responsible for sunburn, while UVA rays penetrate deeper into the skin and contribute to premature aging and, crucially in this context, the darkening of scars.

The Sun Protection Factor (SPF) indicates the level of protection against UVB rays. For scar protection, an SPF of **30 or higher** is generally recommended, with SPF 50 or higher offering even greater protection. It is vital to select "broad-spectrum" products to ensure comprehensive defence.

Application of sunscreen should be a ritual, not an afterthought.

For optimal protection, sunscreen should be applied generously to the scar area at least **15 to 20 minutes before any anticipated sun exposure**. This allows the active ingredients to bind to the skin and form a protective barrier. Crucially, reapplication is key. Sunscreen wears off due to sweat, friction, and simply the passage of time.

Therefore, it needs to be reapplied at least every **two hours**, and more frequently if swimming or sweating heavily. Don't forget to protect areas that might be indirectly exposed, such as the edges of a scar or areas covered by clothing that might shift. The texture of the sunscreen is also a consideration. Many individuals find thicker, cream-based sunscreens to be more effective for direct application on scars, as they tend to stay in place better.

Mineral-based sunscreens, containing zinc oxide and titanium dioxide, are often recommended for sensitive skin and scars, as they sit on the skin's surface and physically block UV rays, making them less likely to cause irritation.

However, sunscreen alone, while essential, may not always be sufficient, especially for individuals who spend extended periods outdoors or have a history of significant sun sensitivity. Therefore, **physical barriers** play an equally important role in protecting scars. **Protective clothing** is an invaluable tool. When possible, opt for garments made from tightly woven fabrics that offer a physical shield against UV radiation. Long-sleeved shirts, long pants, and wide-brimmed hats can significantly reduce the amount of UV light reaching the skin.

For scars on the face, neck, or arms, wearing clothing that covers the scar is the most reliable method of protection. Consider UPF (Ultraviolet Protection Factor) rated clothing for an added layer of assurance, similar to how SPF works for sunscreen.

The simple act of **seeking shade** is another powerful, yet often overlooked, strategy. During peak sun hours, typically between 10 a.m. and 4 p.m., when UV radiation is at its strongest, it is advisable to minimize direct sun exposure. If you are outdoors, try to find shady spots under trees, umbrellas, or awnings.

This is particularly important for individuals who work outdoors or engage in recreational activities that keep them exposed to the sun for long periods.

Planning activities for earlier in the morning or later in the afternoon can also help in avoiding the most intense sun rays.

For scars that are particularly difficult to cover with clothing or sunscreen, such as those on the scalp or on parts of the face not easily shielded, specialized scar care products that incorporate SPF can be a beneficial addition.

These might include silicone sheets or gels with added SPF, or tinted moisturizers with sun protection properties that can help camouflage the scar while offering some protection. It is important to remember that even on cloudy days, UV rays can penetrate cloud cover, so sun protection should be a year-round practice, not just reserved for sunny summer days.

The commitment to sun protection for scars is a long-term investment in preventing what could be years of frustration with discoloration.

While topical treatments and other scar therapies aim to improve the texture and colour of scars, their effectiveness can be significantly undermined by ongoing sun damage. A darkened or lightened scar resulting from sun exposure can be much harder to treat, and in some cases, the changes may be permanent. Therefore, incorporating these simple yet effective sun protection measures into your daily routine is paramount. It's about being proactive, consistent, and informed about how to best safeguard your healing skin. By diligently protecting your scars from the sun, you significantly increase the likelihood of achieving a more even, less conspicuous, and aesthetically pleasing outcome. This consistent effort will pay dividends in the long run, preserving the results of other scar treatments and contributing to your overall skin health and confidence.

Gentle scar massage is a powerful, yet often underutilized, tool in the comprehensive management of scar tissue.

While topical treatments and diligent sun protection form crucial first lines of defence, the mechanical manipulation of scar tissue through massage offers a complementary approach that directly addresses the physical characteristics of a scar: its stiffness, adherence, and potential for restricting movement. This technique empowers individuals with a hands-on method to actively participate in their scar healing journey, fostering a more pliable, less noticeable scar over time. The core principle behind scar massage is to encourage the remodelling of the collagen matrix that forms the scar, breaking down excessive or disorganized fibrous tissue and promoting a more flexible and integrated result.

The benefits of scar massage extend beyond mere cosmetic improvement. By applying gentle, consistent pressure and movement, you can effectively address several key issues that commonly arise with scar formation. One of the most significant advantages is the improvement of **scar mobility and reduction of tightness**. Scar tissue, by its nature, is denser and less elastic than the surrounding healthy skin and underlying tissues. This can lead to a feeling of pulling or tightness, especially when the scar is located over a joint or in an area prone to stretching. Massage helps to gradually lengthen and loosen these inelastic fibres, allowing for a greater range of motion and relieving the discomfort associated with restricted movement. This is particularly important for surgical scars that might be deep and involve underlying muscle or fascia.

Furthermore, scar massage plays a vital role in **enhancing tissue pliability**.

Over time, scar tissue can become hard and somewhat rigid. Massage techniques, when applied correctly, work to soften this hardened tissue, making it feel more like the surrounding skin.

This improved pliability not only contributes to a better aesthetic outcome but also reduces the risk of the scar becoming overly prominent or developing hypertrophic characteristics. The manipulation helps to redistribute collagen fibres, encouraging them to align in a more organized and less haphazard manner, which is the hallmark of mature, well-healed scar tissue.

A crucial mechanism through which scar massage operates is by helping to **break down scar adhesions**. Adhesions are bands of scar tissue that can form between the scar and underlying structures, or even within different layers of the scar itself. These adhesions can significantly restrict movement and cause pain or discomfort. Gentle massage, with its focus on gliding and stretching the tissue, can help to gently separate these adhered layers, restoring a smoother gliding motion between the scar and the tissues beneath it. This can be especially beneficial for scars that feel "stuck" or that cause a pulling sensation with movement.

Another significant benefit is the **improvement of circulation to the scar area**. Scar tissue often has compromised blood supply compared to normal skin. Increased blood flow is essential for delivering oxygen and nutrients needed for tissue repair and remodelling. The gentle pressure and friction from massage can stimulate local blood vessels, increasing circulation in and around the scar. This enhanced vascularity can aid in the delivery of beneficial cells and molecules that promote healthy collagen remodelling and can help to reduce redness or a purplish hue that may be present in newer scars. The increased circulation also helps to flush away waste products, further supporting the healing process.

Finally, scar massage actively **promotes a more organized collagen matrix**. When the skin is injured, the body's primary response is to produce collagen to repair the damage. In the case of scars, this collagen production can sometimes be excessive or disorganized, leading to the visible and palpable characteristics of a scar. Massage acts as a form of controlled mechanical stress, which signals to the fibroblasts (the cells responsible for collagen production) to remodel the existing collagen. This encourages the collagen fibers to align in a more parallel and organized fashion, resulting in a flatter, softer, and less noticeable scar. Think of it as guiding the building blocks of the scar to form a more structured and less rigid framework.

Understanding when to begin scar massage is paramount to ensure safety and maximize effectiveness. Generally, it is recommended to wait until the wound is **fully closed and epithelialized**. This means that there are no open areas, scabs, or oozing. Typically, this is a few days to a week or two after stitches are removed, depending on the wound and the individual's healing rate. Massaging too early, when the wound is still open, can disrupt the healing process, increase the risk of infection, and potentially worsen the scar. Always consult with your healthcare provider or surgeon to determine the optimal time to commence scar massage for your specific situation. They can provide personalized guidance based on the nature of your scar, whether it resulted from surgery, injury, or a dermatological procedure.

Once it is safe to begin, the application of **gentle, consistent pressure** is the cornerstone of effective scar massage. The goal is not to cause pain, but to apply enough pressure to feel a slight stretching or pressure sensation within the scar tissue.

Imagine you are trying to move the scar tissue across the underlying structures without causing discomfort. Start with very light pressure and gradually increase it over time as the scar matures and becomes less sensitive. The pressure should feel firm but yielding, not sharp or digging.

There are several fundamental massage techniques that can be employed for scar softening. One of the most accessible and effective is **circular friction**. With your fingertip or thumb, gently rub the scar in small, concentric circles. You can either move the finger in circles on top of the scar, or you can gently grasp the scar and move the surrounding tissue in circles. The key is to create a gentle gliding or friction motion over the scar tissue. Focus on applying pressure directly to the scar, moving both the scar tissue itself and the tissue around it. This helps to break up adhesions and soften the fibrous bands.

Another valuable technique is **linear stroking or stretching**. With the scar fully released, use your fingertips to gently stroke along the length of the scar, applying a slight stretching pressure. You can also stroke across the width of the scar. The direction of these strokes can be varied.

For instance, if the scar is horizontal, you might stroke vertically over it, gently stretching the skin perpendicular to the scar's orientation. This technique is excellent for lengthening scar tissue and improving its elasticity.

**Cross-friction massage** involves applying pressure perpendicular to the direction of the scar. This can be particularly effective for breaking down adhesions and promoting a more organized collagen matrix.

Use your fingertips to apply firm pressure across the scar, moving back and forth. The sensation should be one of deep pressure and stretching, but it should not be painful.

For deeper scars, or those that feel tethered to underlying structures, a technique involving **pinching and lifting** can be beneficial. Gently pinch the scar tissue between your thumb and forefinger. Then, without letting go, try to gently lift and roll the tissue. This helps to mobilize the scar from the underlying fascia and can release tethered points. Be very gentle with this technique, especially in the initial stages, and only apply enough pressure to feel a slight "give" in the tissue.

When adapting techniques for different scar types and locations, consider the characteristics of the scar and its surroundings. For **flat, superficial scars**, circular friction and linear stroking are often sufficient. For **raised or hypertrophic scars**, which are more prominent and often red, a combination of techniques can be beneficial. Initially, focus on gentle friction to soften the tissue. As the scar matures and becomes less inflamed, you can incorporate more pressure and linear stretching.

For **depressed or atrophic scars**, which appear as indentations, the goal is to stimulate collagen production and improve the underlying tissue support. While massage can help, it might be more beneficial to combine it with other treatments. However, gentle massage can still improve the pliability of the surrounding tissue, which may indirectly improve the appearance of the indentation over time.

When massaging scars located over **joints**, such as elbows, knees, or fingers, extra care is needed. The skin in these areas is naturally more mobile.

Massage should focus on improving the gliding motion of the scar over the joint. Gentle linear strokes parallel and perpendicular to the scar, combined with small circular motions, can help prevent the scar from becoming restricted and impeding movement. Always perform these movements within your comfortable range of motion, and never force the joint.

Scars on the **face** require a delicate approach due to the thinness of the skin and the presence of numerous nerve endings and delicate structures. Use very light pressure and focus on circular motions and gentle linear strokes. Avoid any pulling or tugging that could cause discomfort or damage. The goal is to soften the tissue and improve its elasticity without causing irritation.

For scars on the **neck**, be mindful of the underlying thyroid and carotid arteries. Use very gentle pressure and avoid deep, vigorous massage in this area. Focus on superficial friction and gentle stretching.

For scars on the **trunk**, such as the abdomen or back, you can often apply a bit more pressure, provided it is comfortable. These areas typically have thicker skin and can tolerate more robust massage techniques to break down adhesions and improve tissue pliability.

The importance of **consistency and patience** cannot be overstated when it comes to scar massage. This is not a quick fix. It requires a commitment to regular practice, ideally daily or at least several times a week, to see significant results. Scar remodelling is a slow process that can take months, even years. Initially, you might not notice much difference, but with consistent effort, you will begin to feel the scar becoming softer, more pliable, and less tight.

The duration of each massage session can vary, but aiming for **5-10 minutes per scar, per session** is a good starting point. It is better to do shorter, more frequent sessions than longer, infrequent ones. Listen to your body; if a particular technique or pressure level causes pain, reduce the intensity or discontinue it and consult with your healthcare provider.

Scar massage is a powerful adjunctive therapy that complements other scar management strategies, including topical treatments and sun protection. It empowers you to take an active role in improving the appearance and function of your scar. By understanding the principles behind scar massage, learning the appropriate techniques, and committing to consistent practice, you can significantly contribute to a more favourable scar outcome, leading to improved comfort, mobility, and aesthetic satisfaction. It is a testament to the body's ability to heal and remodel, and with gentle guidance through massage, we can help steer that process towards the best possible result.

While we usually think of light just for seeing, certain types of light can actually "feed" our cells. LED Light Therapy (also called Photobiomodulation) uses specific colours of light to help the skin repair itself after an injury. Energy for Cells: Think of the light as a battery charger. When red or near-infrared light hits the skin, it goes deep into the cells and gives them a boost of energy (ATP). This extra energy helps the cells work faster to fix the damage. Smoothing the Texture: One of the biggest problems with scars is that the body sometimes rushes the repair, creating thick or bumpy skin. LED light tells the skin to produce collagen in a more organized way. This makes the scar flatter, softer, and more flexible. Calming the Redness: LED light is excellent at "putting out the fire" of inflammation.

It reduces the angry red or purple colour of new scars and helps stop the itching and tightness that often come with healing.

Simple and Safe: Unlike surgery or harsh chemicals, this treatment is completely painless. You simply sit under the light for about 10 to 20 minutes. Over a few weeks, the scar begins to blend in better with the healthy skin around it.

In short, LED light doesn't just hide a scar—it helps the body do a better job of rebuilding the skin from the inside out.

Not all light is the same. To treat a scar effectively, we use different wavelengths that reach different depths of the skin:

Red Light (630–660 nm) – The Surface Smoother:

This is the go-to colour for most scars. It stays in the upper layers of the skin to boost collagen and elastin. It's best for fading the "angry" red colour of new scars and smoothing out the surface texture.

Near-Infrared Light (830–850 nm) – The Deep Healer:

This light is invisible to the human eye because it travels much deeper—reaching the muscles and deep tissue. It is perfect for thick, tough scars or scars from deep surgery. It helps soften the "hardness" (induration) of a scar and reduces deep-seated inflammation.

Blue Light (415–470 nm) – The Acne Scar Specialist:

Blue light is famous for killing bacteria, making it great for preventing scars while you still have active breakouts. Recent studies also suggest it might help stop keloids (thick, raised scars) from growing too large by slowing down overactive skin cells.

# CHAPTER FOUR

## Advanced Treatments: Medical Interventions for Scar Revision

Corticosteroid injections represent a cornerstone in the medical management of problematic scar tissue, particularly those scars that are characterized by excessive bulk and inflammation, such as hypertrophic scars and keloids. These interventions harness the potent anti-inflammatory and immunosuppressive properties of corticosteroids to directly target the overactive fibroblasts and excessive collagen deposition that define these raised scars. By modulating the cellular and molecular processes involved in scar formation, intralesional corticosteroid injections offer a significant pathway towards softening, flattening, and ultimately improving the appearance and comfort of keloidal and hypertrophic scarring.

Steroid injections work by targeting the two main things that make a scar thick: inflammation and overgrowth.

When the medicine is injected into the scar, it blocks the chemicals that cause swelling and irritation.

At the same time, it tells the skin's "building cells" to stop making so much collagen.

By calming the inflammation and slowing down new tissue growth, the scar becomes flatter, softer, and less noticeable.

The procedure itself is typically performed in a physician's office and is considered minimally invasive. After the treatment area is cleansed, a fine-gauge needle is used to inject a dilute solution of a corticosteroid, most commonly triamcinolone acetonide, directly into the raised portion of the scar. The volume and concentration of the corticosteroid are carefully determined based on the size, thickness, and location of the scar. Patients may experience a brief, sharp sensation during the injection, and some temporary discomfort or a burning feeling may follow, which usually subsides within a few hours. The frequency of injections is highly variable and depends on the scar's response to treatment. Initially, treatments may be administered every 4 to 6 weeks. As the scar begins to flatten and soften, the intervals between injections may be extended. Some individuals may require only a few injections to achieve satisfactory results, while others with more extensive or recalcitrant scarring might benefit from a longer course of treatment. The goal is to achieve a gradual improvement rather than an immediate dramatic change, allowing the body's natural remodelling processes to be guided by the therapeutic intervention.

The expected outcomes from corticosteroid injections are often quite favourable, particularly for hypertrophic scars and keloids. A significant reduction in scar height and thickness is commonly observed, leading to a flatter, less protuberant scar. The associated redness or purplish hue often associated with active, raised scars tends to diminish as the inflammation subsides, contributing to a more subtle appearance. Patients frequently report a decrease in scar-related symptoms, such as itching, tenderness, and pain, which can significantly improve their quality of life.

The improved texture and pliability of the scar tissue are also notable benefits, making the scar feel softer and less restrictive. While complete scar elimination is rarely achievable, the goal is to render the scar less noticeable and more integrated with the surrounding skin, minimizing its psychological and physical impact.

However, like any medical intervention, corticosteroid injections are associated with potential side effects and limitations. One of the most common adverse effects is iatrogenic atrophy, or skin thinning, at the injection site. This occurs due to the inhibitory effect of corticosteroids on collagen synthesis in normal skin as well as scar tissue. This thinning can sometimes lead to a depressed or indented appearance in the treated area, particularly with repeated or high-dose injections. Another potential side effect is hypopigmentation, a lightening of the skin in the treated area. This is usually temporary but can be persistent in some individuals, creating a noticeable contrast with the surrounding skin. In some instances, hyperpigmentation (darkening of the skin) can also occur, though less commonly. Another observed phenomenon is the development of telangiectasias, which are small, dilated blood vessels that can appear on the surface of the treated scar, giving it a somewhat mottled or "spiderweb" appearance. Although rare, systemic absorption of corticosteroids can lead to side effects such as adrenal suppression, particularly with very frequent or high-dose injections, though this is seldom a concern with intralesional administration for scar treatment. Infection at the injection site is also a risk, though minimized by sterile techniques. Furthermore, it is important to note that corticosteroid injections are generally less effective for atrophic or depressed scars, where the goal is to stimulate collagen, not suppress it.

In such cases, other treatment modalities are often preferred. Careful patient selection and meticulous technique are paramount to maximize the benefits of corticosteroid injections while minimizing the risks of adverse effects. Regular follow-up and communication with the treating physician are essential to monitor progress and manage any untoward reactions.

Laser treatments use precise beams of light to fix how a scar looks and feels. Unlike surgery, lasers use energy to target specific layers of the skin without damaging the healthy tissue around them.

The laser creates a "controlled injury" that signals your body to heal itself. This process breaks down old, lumpy tissue and triggers the growth of new, smoother skin. It also shrinks the tiny blood vessels that make scars look red. Because lasers can be adjusted for different skin types and scar depths, they are highly effective at flattening raised scars, filling in pitted ones, and fading discoloration.

The landscape of laser treatments for scars can be broadly categorized into two primary approaches: ablative and non-ablative.

Each category employs distinct mechanisms of action to achieve scar improvement, and their selection depends on the nature of the scar and the desired treatment intensity.

**Ablative Laser Resurfacing:** This category represents the more aggressive end of the laser scar treatment spectrum.

Ablative lasers, such as the carbon dioxide (CO2) laser and the Erbium:YAG (Er:YAG) laser, work by precisely removing thin layers of the epidermis and upper dermis.

Think of it as a controlled vaporization of the skin's surface.

The energy delivered by these lasers is absorbed by the water molecules within the skin tissue, causing it to heat up rapidly and turn into vapor, essentially ablating (removing) the outermost layers of the scar. This physical removal of damaged and disorganized tissue serves several crucial purposes. Firstly, it eliminates superficial textural irregularities, smoothing out the uneven contours that are often characteristic of scars. Secondly, and perhaps most importantly, the controlled injury induced by the laser beam triggers a robust wound healing response. This response involves the activation of fibroblasts, the cells responsible for producing collagen. However, in the context of laser resurfacing, this activation leads to the deposition of new, more organized collagen, gradually replacing the older, haphazardly laid-down collagen of the scar tissue. This process of neocollagenesis is central to improving the scar's texture, reducing its depth, and enhancing its overall pliability. The depth of ablation can be precisely controlled by adjusting the laser's energy settings, the density of the laser pulses (how closely packed they are), and the number of passes the physician makes over the scar. This meticulous control allows for tailoring the treatment to the specific needs of the scar, from mild textural imperfections to deeper, more significant depressions.

The CO2 laser, with its wavelength of 10,600 nm, has a high affinity for water and thus penetrates deeply into the skin, leading to significant ablation and thermal coagulation.

This deep penetration and thermal effect are highly effective for treating deep wrinkles, severe acne scarring, and other textural irregularities. The heat generated not only vaporizes tissue but also stimulates collagen remodelling far below the surface.

However, the deeper penetration and more significant thermal effect of the CO2 laser also translate to longer downtime and a higher risk of side effects, such as post-inflammatory hyperpigmentation, especially in individuals with darker skin tones.

The Er:YAG laser, operating at a wavelength of 2,940 nm, is also highly absorbed by water but has a shallower penetration depth compared to the CO2 laser.

This makes it a gentler option, primarily targeting the epidermis and the superficial dermis. Er:YAG lasers are excellent for treating superficial textural issues, fine lines, and less severe scarring.

Because they cause less thermal damage to the surrounding tissue, they generally result in shorter recovery times and a reduced risk of pigmentary complications compared to CO2 lasers.

Many modern ablative laser systems offer a "fractional" mode, which will be discussed in more detail later, but the underlying principle of ablating tissue remains the core of their function.

The procedure for ablative laser resurfacing typically begins with thorough cleansing of the treatment area and the application of a topical anaesthetic cream to minimize discomfort.

Many practitioners also administer local anaesthetic injections or use a cooling device during the procedure.

The laser handpiece is then moved over the scar tissue in a systematic pattern, delivering controlled energy pulses.

Patients often describe a sensation of heat or snapping, depending on the anaesthesia used.

After the procedure, the treated area will appear red and may be swollen, similar to a sunburn.

It will likely be sensitive to the touch and may ooze serous fluid. Strict post-operative care is crucial, involving regular cleansing, the application of soothing ointments, and diligent sun protection to prevent complications and optimize healing. Downtime can range from several days to a couple of weeks, depending on the depth of the treatment and the individual's healing capacity.

During this period, the skin will undergo a process of re-epithelialization, where new skin cells form and cover the treated area. The results of ablative laser resurfacing can be dramatic, with significant improvements in scar texture, smoothness, and a reduction in depth. The new collagen produced can take several months to fully mature, so the full benefits of the treatment may not be apparent for up to six months or even longer.

**Non-Ablative Laser Resurfacing:** In contrast to ablative lasers, non-ablative lasers work by delivering thermal energy into the dermis without vaporizing the surface layers of the skin. The primary goal of non-ablative lasers is to heat the underlying tissue, specifically the collagen, to stimulate a wound healing response and promote the production of new, healthier collagen.

This approach bypasses the epidermal injury associated with ablative lasers, which translates to significantly shorter downtime and a lower risk of adverse effects, particularly pigmentary changes.

While they may not offer the dramatic textural smoothing of ablative lasers for very deep scars, non-ablative lasers are excellent for improving mild to moderate textural irregularities, fine lines, and promoting overall skin rejuvenation.

A prominent example of a non-ablative laser used for scar treatment is the fractional laser. Fractional laser technology, which can be either ablative or non-ablative, revolutionizes resurfacing by treating the skin in a microscopic pattern. Instead of treating the entire surface of the scar, fractional lasers create thousands of microscopic treatment zones (MTZs) within the skin, leaving the surrounding tissue intact. These untreated areas act as reservoirs of healthy cells, which can migrate into the treated zones, significantly accelerating the healing process. This "fractional" approach is what allows for effective collagen stimulation and tissue remodelling with considerably less downtime and fewer risks than traditional, fully ablative resurfacing.

**Non-ablative fractional lasers**, such as those employing wavelengths like 1540 nm (e.g., Erbium:Glass laser) or 1440 nm, deliver controlled heat into the dermis within these MTZs. This heat stimulates fibroblasts to produce new collagen and elastin, leading to a gradual improvement in scar texture, firmness, and smoothness. These lasers are particularly effective for improving the appearance of acne scars, surgical scars, and other types of textural irregularities that are not excessively deep. The benefits are seen over time as collagen remodelling occurs. Patients typically require a series of treatments, often spaced several weeks apart, to achieve optimal results. The downtime associated with non-ablative fractional laser treatment is generally minimal, often consisting of mild redness and some swelling that subsides within a day or two. The procedure itself is usually well-tolerated, with a sensation of warmth or mild prickling, and topical anaesthetics can be used to enhance comfort.

Beyond general resurfacing, specific laser modalities are tailored to address particular characteristics of scar tissue.

**Pulsed Dye Lasers (PDL):** These lasers are exceptionally effective at targeting the redness and vascularity often associated with newer, actively healing scars, as well as hypertrophic scars and keloids. PDLs, such as the Vbeam or Cynergy systems, operate at wavelengths around 585 nm or 595 nm, which are highly absorbed by hemoglobins, the molecule responsible for the red colour of blood. When the PDL light energy is absorbed by the abnormal blood vessels within the scar tissue, it causes them to heat up and selectively coagulate, or collapse.

This process leads to a reduction in redness and can help to flatten raised scars by reducing their vascular supply. PDLs are generally considered safe and effective for most skin types, although caution is advised with darker skin tones due to the potential for pigmentary changes.

The procedure involves delivering short pulses of light energy to the scar, and patients typically experience a sensation of stinging or snapping. Bruising is a common side effect that usually resolves within a week to ten days.

Multiple treatment sessions, typically spaced 4-8 weeks apart, are usually required to achieve significant improvement in scar redness and thickness. PDLs can also help to alleviate associated symptoms like itching and tenderness in some scars.

**Alexandrite and Diode Lasers:** Lasers operating at longer wavelengths, such as the Alexandrite laser (755 nm) and diode lasers (800-810 nm), can also be utilized for scar revision, particularly for addressing pigmentary issues and hair removal in scarred areas.

While not primarily ablative or designed for deep collagen remodelling like CO2 or Er:YAG lasers, their energy can penetrate the dermis to some extent and may contribute to subtle textural improvements over time, especially in combination with other treatments.

Their efficacy in scar revision is often secondary to their primary applications, but they can play a role in managing specific aspects of scar appearance.

**Fractional Non-Ablative Lasers and Their Applications:** As mentioned earlier, fractional non-ablative lasers have become a cornerstone in modern scar management due to their favourable balance of efficacy and safety. Their ability to create microscopic zones of thermal injury while preserving surrounding healthy tissue leads to robust collagen stimulation and remodelling with minimal downtime. For atrophic scars, such as those resulting from acne or chickenpox, fractional non-ablative lasers are invaluable. They work by stimulating the production of new collagen in the dermal layer, effectively "plumping up" the depressed areas and improving the overall smoothness of the skin. The process is gradual, with collagen synthesis continuing for months after treatment, leading to progressive improvement.

For hypertrophic scars and keloids, fractional lasers can also be beneficial, though often in conjunction with other therapies like corticosteroid injections or silicone sheeting. The controlled thermal injury can help to break down the excess collagen that characterizes these raised scars and stimulate a more organized deposition of new collagen. Furthermore, fractional laser treatments can help to improve the texture and colour of these scars over time, making them less noticeable.

The application of fractional lasers is highly versatile. They can be used on a variety of scar types, including acne scars, surgical scars, traumatic scars, and even stretch marks (striae). The treatment parameters are adjusted based on the depth of the scar, the patient's skin type, and the desired outcome. Typically, a series of 3-5 treatments, spaced 4-6 weeks apart, are recommended for optimal results. Post-treatment care usually involves applying a soothing moisturizer and diligent sun protection. While downtime is minimal, some redness and mild swelling may persist for a day or two. The gradual nature of collagen remodelling means that the full benefits of fractional laser treatments may not be visible for several months, and touch-up treatments may be necessary to maintain results.

The patient experience with laser scar revision is an important consideration. Before undergoing any laser treatment, a thorough consultation with a qualified dermatologist or plastic surgeon is essential. During this consultation, the physician will assess the scar tissue, discuss the patient's goals and expectations, and determine the most appropriate laser modality or combination of treatments. It is crucial for patients to understand that scar revision is often a process, and multiple treatment sessions may be required to achieve the desired outcome. The physician will also discuss the potential risks and benefits associated with each type of laser, including the possibility of pain, swelling, redness, bruising, pigmentary changes

(hypopigmentation or hyperpigmentation), and infection. Contraindications, such as active infections, certain medications, or a history of keloid formation in response to laser treatment, will also be reviewed.

The actual laser treatment procedure varies depending on the type of laser used. For ablative lasers, the skin is typically numbed with a topical anaesthetic cream for 30-60 minutes prior to the procedure. For non-ablative lasers, topical anaesthesia may also be used, or a cooling device may be employed during treatment to enhance comfort. During the procedure, the laser handpiece is guided over the scar tissue, delivering controlled energy. Patients may experience sensations of warmth, tingling, or mild stinging. After the treatment, the skin will appear red and may be swollen, similar to a sunburn. Post-treatment care is critical for optimal healing and to minimize the risk of complications. This typically involves cleansing the treated area gently, applying prescribed ointments or creams to promote healing and prevent infection, and strictly adhering to sun avoidance and the use of broad-spectrum sunscreen.

Downtime, a crucial factor for patients, differs significantly between ablative and non-ablative lasers. Ablative laser resurfacing involves significant downtime, often ranging from 7 to 14 days, during which the skin peels and re-epithelializes.

During this period, patients may need to stay home from work and avoid strenuous activities. Non-ablative laser treatments, including fractional non-ablative lasers, have much shorter downtime, typically only a day or two of mild redness and swelling that can often be concealed with makeup.

The results of laser scar revision can be transformative, but it's important to have realistic expectations. Complete scar elimination is rarely achievable. Instead, the goal is to improve the scar's appearance, making it less noticeable and more integrated with the surrounding skin.

Significant improvements in texture, colour, and smoothness can be achieved, leading to enhanced self-confidence and a better quality of life for the patient. The long-term results depend on the individual's healing response, the type and severity of the scar, and the number and type of treatments performed.

Ongoing maintenance treatments may be recommended for some individuals to sustain the achieved results.

As technology continues to advance, laser therapy offers an increasingly refined and effective approach to scar revision, providing hope for those seeking to minimize the impact of scarring on their appearance and well-being.

The careful selection of laser technology, precise application, and diligent post-treatment care are paramount to achieving the best possible outcomes in the journey of scar rejuvenation.

**Microneedling**, a minimally invasive procedure also referred to as collagen induction therapy or derma rolling, has rapidly gained prominence as a valuable tool in the comprehensive management of scar tissue. Unlike laser therapies that employ focused light energy, microneedling harnesses the body's inherent regenerative capabilities through the creation of precisely controlled micro-injuries. The fundamental principle underpinning this technique lies in its ability to stimulate the skin's natural wound healing cascade, thereby orchestrating a symphony of cellular responses that ultimately lead to dermal remodelling and improved scar appearance.

The process begins with the utilization of a device equipped with an array of ultra-fine, sterile needles. These needles can be integrated into a manual roller, a stamping device, or an automated pen-like instrument.

As the device is passed over the scar tissue, these microscopic needles penetrate the epidermis and superficial dermis, creating a multitude of minuscule, intentional puncture wounds. These seemingly minor injuries, often measuring between 0.5 and 2.5 millimetres in depth, are the catalysts for a profound biological response. Crucially, these perforations are significantly smaller than those inflicted by traditional surgical procedures or even the thermal injury from certain lasers. This controlled micro-trauma is interpreted by the skin not as damage requiring repair in the conventional sense, but rather as a signal to initiate an accelerated healing and regeneration process.

Microneedling works by tricking your skin into healing itself. When the tiny needles create microscopic holes, your body immediately releases "growth factors"—natural signals that tell your skin to start repairing. These signals wake up special cells called fibroblasts. These cells act like a construction crew, building new collagen, which is the protein that gives your skin its strength and smoothness. By creating this fresh layer of collagen, microneedling helps fill in and rebuild the uneven areas caused by scarring.

Beyond collagen, the production of elastin, another vital protein responsible for skin's suppleness and ability to recoil, is also upregulated by microneedling. Scar tissue is often characterized by a disorganized and diminished elastin network, contributing to its stiffness and altered texture. By stimulating elastogenesis, microneedling helps to restore some of the lost elasticity, making the scar tissue feel softer and more pliable. The newly synthesized collagen and elastin fibres are laid down in a more organized and parallel fashion compared to the haphazard arrangement typically found in mature scar tissue.

This improved structural organization contributes significantly to the textural refinement of the scar.

The efficacy of microneedling is particularly notable for atrophic scars, which are characterized by a depressed or indented appearance. These types of scars, often the result of acne, chickenpox, or superficial trauma, occur when there is insufficient collagen and elastin production during the initial healing phase, leading to a loss of underlying dermal volume. Microneedling effectively addresses this by stimulating the body to lay down new collagen and elastin in these depleted areas. As the dermis is rebuilt from within, the depressed contours of the atrophic scar begin to fill in, leading to a smoother, more even skin surface. The process is not instantaneous; rather, it unfolds over weeks and months as the new collagen and elastin mature and integrate into the existing dermal matrix.

While microneedling is most widely recognized for its benefits in atrophic scarring, it also demonstrates considerable promise in improving the appearance of certain hypertrophic scars and even keloids, although its role in these more complex scar types is often as an adjunct therapy. Hypertrophic scars are raised, thickened scars that remain within the boundaries of the original wound, while keloids are an even more aggressive form that extend beyond the original wound margins. In these cases, microneedling can help to break down the excess, disorganized collagen that characterizes these raised scars. The controlled micro-injury and the subsequent release of growth factors can stimulate the remodelling of mature collagen and encourage the deposition of newer, more organized collagen, potentially leading to a flattening and softening of the scar tissue over time.

However, for significant hypertrophic scarring or keloids, microneedling is frequently combined with other treatments, such as intralesional corticosteroid injections, silicone gel sheeting, or even laser therapy, to achieve optimal results.

The procedure itself is generally well-tolerated and can be performed in an outpatient clinical setting. Prior to treatment, the targeted scar area is thoroughly cleansed to minimize the risk of infection. Topical anaesthetic creams, typically containing lidocaine or a combination of lidocaine and prilocaine, are applied to the skin and allowed to take effect for approximately 30 to 60 minutes. This significantly numbs the surface layers of the skin, rendering the procedure comfortable for most patients. During the treatment, the microneedling device is passed over the scar in a systematic pattern, ensuring uniform coverage. Patients often report a sensation of mild pressure or a prickling feeling, but with adequate anaesthesia, pain is usually minimal. The depth of the needles is carefully selected by the practitioner based on the type of scar, its location, and the patient's skin thickness. For delicate areas or very superficial scars, shorter needles may be used, while deeper or more fibrotic scars might necessitate longer needle lengths to reach the reticular dermis where collagen remodelling is most effectively stimulated.

Following the microneedling procedure, the treated skin will typically appear red and may exhibit mild swelling, akin to a mild sunburn.

This inflammatory response is a natural and expected part of the healing process.

Patients are usually advised to keep the area clean and to apply a soothing, hypoallergenic moisturizer.

The redness and swelling usually subside within 24 to 72 hours.

Unlike ablative laser resurfacing, which involves the removal of skin layers and can result in significant downtime and crusting, microneedling is associated with much shorter recovery periods. Most patients can resume their normal daily activities, including work, within a day or two after the procedure, with minimal visible signs of treatment beyond transient redness. Diligent sun protection is paramount during the healing phase and ongoing, as newly formed collagen can be more susceptible to photodamage.

The results of microneedling are not immediate. The true benefits emerge as the body's collagen and elastin production continues over several weeks and months. Patients typically require a series of treatments to achieve significant and lasting improvement in scar appearance. The number of sessions needed varies depending on the severity and type of scar, as well as the individual's response to treatment. Generally, a series of three to six microneedling sessions, spaced four to six weeks apart, is recommended to allow sufficient time for collagen remodelling between treatments. Some patients may benefit from maintenance treatments at longer intervals to sustain the improvements.

One of the significant advantages of microneedling is its versatility and the potential for synergistic combination therapies. The micro-channels created by the needles can serve as conduits for the topical application of active ingredients, enhancing their penetration into the dermis. This has led to the development and widespread use of "collagen induction therapy" in conjunction with specific serums or solutions. For scar revision, serums containing growth factors, hyaluronic acid, peptides, or even certain antioxidants can be applied immediately after microneedling to further support the healing and regenerative processes.

A particularly powerful enhancement to microneedling is its combination with radiofrequency (RF) energy. Radiofrequency microneedling devices deliver RF energy through the needles into the deeper layers of the dermis simultaneously as the needles create micro-injuries. This dual action offers a significant advantage: the microneedling creates the pathways for the RF energy to penetrate more deeply and effectively, while the RF energy itself heats the tissue, leading to more profound collagen contraction and neocollagenesis. The thermal energy delivered by RF not only stimulates fibroblasts but also causes immediate tightening of existing collagen fibres, contributing to a firmer and smoother appearance of the scar. This combination therapy is particularly effective for deeper atrophic scars and can yield more dramatic results than microneedling alone, often with comparable or slightly increased downtime.

Another increasingly popular adjunct to microneedling is the use of platelet-rich plasma (PRP). PRP is derived from the patient's own blood, which is drawn and then processed in a centrifuge to concentrate the platelets. Platelets are rich in growth factors, and when applied topically or infused into the micro-channels created by microneedling, they can significantly amplify the regenerative response. The concentrated growth factors in PRP further stimulate fibroblast activity, enhance collagen synthesis, and promote tissue repair. The combination of microneedling with PRP, often referred to as "vampire facial" for general rejuvenation, can be highly beneficial for scar revision by providing a potent cocktail of biological signals to accelerate and optimize the healing and remodelling process.

This approach leverages the body's own regenerative potential to its fullest extent, offering a natural yet powerful method for scar improvement.

Microneedling is generally considered safe for most skin types, including darker skin tones, which can be at higher risk of post-inflammatory hyperpigmentation with some other resurfacing techniques like ablative lasers. The controlled nature of the micro-injuries and the absence of significant thermal or ablative damage minimize the risk of pigmentary alterations. However, as with any procedure, there are potential, albeit rare, side effects such as infection, persistent redness, or scarring, particularly if the procedure is not performed under sterile conditions or if post-care instructions are not followed diligently. A thorough consultation with a qualified healthcare professional is essential to assess suitability, discuss potential risks and benefits, and tailor the treatment plan to the individual's specific scar characteristics and skin type.

The ongoing evolution of microneedling technology, including advanced device designs and the integration with other modalities like RF and PRP, continues to expand its role as a cornerstone therapy in the multidisciplinary approach to scar revision.

Chemical peels and dermabrasion represent two distinct yet complementary approaches to scar revision, both fundamentally relying on the principle of controlled exfoliation to reveal smoother, more uniform skin. While microneedling stimulates the skin's intrinsic healing cascade from within, these methods work from the surface downwards, carefully abrading or dissolving superficial layers of the epidermis and dermis to diminish the visibility of imperfections.

Their efficacy is often most pronounced in addressing superficial textural irregularities, mild discoloration, and shallow atrophic scarring where the depth of the scar is amenable to surface-level remodelling.

Chemical peels, a cornerstone of dermatological and aesthetic treatments for decades, employ the application of specific acidic solutions to the skin. These solutions create a controlled injury to the epidermis and, depending on the depth of the peel and the type of acid used, the upper layers of the dermis. This controlled wounding triggers a natural regenerative response, accelerating cell turnover and prompting the skin to shed its damaged outer layers. The primary goal is to remove the damaged, irregular, or discoloured skin cells that contribute to the scar's appearance and to stimulate the production of new, healthier skin cells beneath. The spectrum of chemical peels ranges from very superficial, which affect only the stratum corneum (the outermost layer of the epidermis), to medium-depth and deep peels, which penetrate further into the dermis. For scar revision, particularly for superficial atrophic scars or post-inflammatory hyperpigmentation associated with scarring, superficial to medium-depth peels are generally the modalities of choice.

Superficial peels commonly utilize agents such as alpha-hydroxy acids (AHAs) like glycolic acid or lactic acid, or beta-hydroxy acids (BHAs) like salicylic acid. These peels work by dissolving the intercellular "glue" that holds dead skin cells together, facilitating their sloughing off. Glycolic acid, with its small molecular size, can penetrate the epidermis efficiently, promoting rapid cell turnover and revealing brighter, smoother skin. Lactic acid, being larger, has a more hydrating effect and is often preferred for individuals with sensitive skin.

Salicylic acid, a lipophilic acid, is particularly effective for oily or acne-prone skin and can penetrate pores, making it beneficial for acne scars that involve clogged pores or residual inflammation. These superficial peels typically result in mild redness, flaking, or peeling over a few days and require minimal downtime. They are excellent for improving mild textural irregularities and superficial discoloration that may accompany certain types of scarring, such as mild post-acne marks.

Medium-depth peels extend their reach into the papillary dermis, the upper layer of the dermis just beneath the epidermis. Trichloroacetic acid (TCA) is a commonly used agent for medium-depth peels, often in concentrations ranging from 35% to 50%. Phenol is another agent used for deeper peels, though it is less commonly employed for general scar revision due to its more aggressive nature and higher risk profile. Medium-depth TCA peels create a more significant controlled injury, leading to more substantial exfoliation and a more pronounced regenerative response. They are particularly effective in addressing more significant textural changes, shallow to moderate atrophic scars, and persistent hyperpigmentation or hypopigmentation that superficial peels cannot fully correct. The downtime associated with medium-depth peels is longer than superficial peels, typically involving several days to a week of redness, swelling, and peeling, with a noticeable period of skin sensitivity and potential for temporary pigmentary changes.

The procedure for a chemical peel is relatively straightforward, though it demands precision and adherence to safety protocols. Before the peel, the skin is thoroughly cleansed and degreased to ensure uniform penetration of the acidic solution.

The chosen chemical agent is then carefully applied to the treatment area using a brush, gauze, or cotton-tipped applicator. The patient may experience a warming or stinging sensation as the acid penetrates the skin, which can be managed with cooling measures such as a fan. The duration of acid contact is carefully controlled, and neutralization or removal of the agent is performed once the desired endpoint is achieved, often indicated by erythema (redness) or a frosted appearance of the skin. Post-peel care is critical and typically involves the application of bland emollients, sun protection, and sometimes prescribed topical agents to aid healing and prevent complications.

While chemical peels are generally safe, they are not without risks. Superficial peels carry a low risk of complications, primarily limited to transient irritation or dryness. Medium-depth peels, however, carry a higher potential for side effects, including prolonged redness, swelling, infection, and more significantly, pigmentary alterations. Post-inflammatory hyperpigmentation (PIH), where the skin darkens in the treated area, is a particular concern, especially in individuals with darker skin types. Conversely, hypopigmentation (lightening of the skin) can also occur. Scarring is a rare but possible complication, particularly if the peel is too deep, improperly applied, or if post-care instructions are not followed meticulously. Therefore, chemical peels should only be performed by trained and experienced practitioners in appropriate settings.

Dermabrasion, in contrast to chemical peels, is a mechanical form of exfoliation. It involves the use of a high-speed rotary instrument, typically equipped with a wire brush or a diamond fraise, to "sand" or abrade the skin's surface.

This process literally removes the outermost layers of the epidermis and papillary dermis, much like sanding wood to smooth out imperfections. Dermabrasion is a more aggressive procedure than most superficial peels and is capable of reaching deeper layers of the dermis, depending on the skill of the operator and the aggressiveness of the technique employed.

The primary indication for dermabrasion in scar revision includes atrophic scars, particularly those with irregular borders or textural irregularities. It can also be effective for ice-pick acne scars, which are deep, narrow, and pitted scars, as well as for superficial burns or surgical scars where there is significant textural disruption. The mechanical removal of the scarred tissue and the underlying layers promotes a healing response that leads to the deposition of new collagen and elastin in a more organized fashion, smoothing out the contours of the scar. The depth to which the skin is abraded is carefully controlled by the practitioner, aiming to remove the abnormal tissue while minimizing the risk of creating a new scar.

The dermabrasion procedure is typically performed under local anaesthesia, often combined with intravenous sedation for patient comfort, especially if larger areas are being treated or if deeper abrasion is planned. The skin is cleansed, and the chosen abrasive instrument is applied with consistent pressure and technique over the scar tissue. Patients often describe a "grinding" or "scraping" sensation, and topical anaesthetic creams are crucial for managing discomfort. The practitioner meticulously works over the scarred area, removing layers of skin until the desired level of improvement is achieved. The treated area will appear raw and bleeding after the procedure.

The recovery period following dermabrasion is generally longer and more involved than that of chemical peels. Immediately after the procedure, the treated area will be covered with a sterile dressing to protect the exposed dermis. Patients will experience significant redness, swelling, and oozing for the first few days. A crust or scab will form over the treated area, which will gradually dry and then peel off over one to two weeks. During this healing phase, diligent wound care is essential to prevent infection and promote optimal healing. Patients are advised to keep the area clean, apply prescribed topical ointments, and avoid any friction or trauma to the healing skin. Sun avoidance is critical, as the newly formed skin is highly susceptible to photodamage and hyperpigmentation.

Potential risks associated with dermabrasion include infection, prolonged redness, swelling, and blistering. As with chemical peels, pigmentary changes, both hyperpigmentation and hypopigmentation, are significant concerns, particularly in individuals with darker skin tones. Scarring is also a risk, especially if the abrasion is too deep or if healing is compromised.

The mechanical nature of the procedure can sometimes lead to a smoother, albeit lighter, appearance of the treated skin compared to the surrounding skin, creating a subtle contrast.

The suitability of both chemical peels and dermabrasion for scar revision is highly dependent on the type, depth, and age of the scar, as well as the patient's skin type and individual healing characteristics. Superficial atrophic scars, acne scars with shallow depressions, and scars with significant discoloration or textural irregularity are generally the best candidates.

Older, more mature scars may be less responsive than newer ones, as their collagen structure has become more established and fibrotic. Individuals with active acne or infection in the treatment area, or those with a history of keloid formation, may not be ideal candidates or may require a modified approach.

It is crucial to understand that neither chemical peels nor dermabrasion are typically standalone solutions for all types of scars, particularly deep or hypertrophic scars.

For severe scarring, they are often used as adjunctive therapies, combined with other modalities such as microneedling, laser resurfacing, surgical scar revision, or corticosteroid injections.

The choice between a chemical peel and dermabrasion, or a combination of treatments, will be determined by a thorough evaluation by a qualified dermatologist or plastic surgeon who can assess the scar characteristics, consider the patient's goals, and recommend the most appropriate and safest treatment plan.

The overarching aim of these exfoliation techniques is to meticulously resurface the skin, diminishing the textural and pigmentary discrepancies that scar tissue introduces, thereby restoring a more harmonious and aesthetically pleasing skin surface.

The success of these procedures hinges on careful patient selection, precise execution by the practitioner, and diligent post-treatment care to optimize healing and minimize complications, ultimately leading to a smoother, more refined skin appearance.

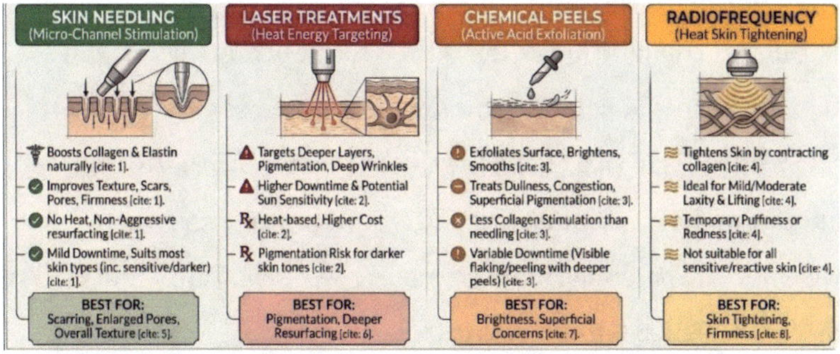


Surgical scar revision represents a distinct category of intervention, reserved for those instances where less invasive methods like chemical peels, dermabrasion, or microneedling have proven insufficient or are simply not indicated. It is a deliberate, often more involved, approach to correcting scars that present significant aesthetic or functional challenges.

The fundamental principle underlying surgical revision is the complete removal of the problematic scar tissue and its replacement with a new incision that, ideally, heals into a less noticeable line.

This technique is not about eradicating scarring entirely – a feat currently beyond our capabilities – but rather about transforming a conspicuous, undesirable scar into one that is more subtle, better positioned, or less disruptive to the skin's natural contours and functionality.

The decision to proceed with surgical scar revision is typically made when a scar is characterized by several undesirable attributes.

These include excessive width, where the scar tissue has spread out, creating a broad and noticeable mark.

Another common indication is a scar that is poorly aligned with the natural lines of tension in the skin, often referred to as "relaxed skin tension lines" (RSTLs). Scars that run perpendicular to these lines are under constant tension and are therefore more prone to widening and becoming more prominent over time. Furthermore, scars that are depressed (atrophic) to a degree that cannot be corrected by surface treatments, or those that are raised and hypertrophic or keloidal beyond what can be managed with injections, may also warrant surgical consideration. Functional impairments, such as scar contractures that restrict movement around a joint, eyelid, or lip, are critical reasons for surgical intervention, as the primary goal in these cases shifts from pure aesthetics to restoring normal function. Irregularity of the scar edges, or a scar that has developed a problematic texture, can also be addressed surgically.

The cornerstone of surgical scar revision is **scar excision and direct closure**. This is perhaps the most straightforward and commonly employed surgical technique. In this procedure, the entire existing scar is meticulously removed with a scalpel. The edges of the wound are then carefully brought together and closed with sutures. The goal of this direct closure is to create a new, thin line of scar tissue that lies along the RSTLs or is strategically positioned to be less visible.

Surgeons will carefully assess the direction of skin tension and the orientation of the scar before making the incision. Often, the scar is excised in an elliptical shape, allowing for tension-free closure.

The choice of sutures, their placement, and the technique used are critical for minimizing tension on the wound edges, which is paramount for achieving a fine, linear scar. This method is most effective for narrower scars or those that can be closed with minimal stretching of the surrounding skin. If a scar is too wide or its removal creates excessive tension upon closure, simple direct closure may result in a new scar that is as wide or even wider than the original. In such instances, alternative surgical techniques become necessary.

When a scar is too wide to allow for tension-free direct closure, or when the underlying tissue is insufficient, a **skin graft** may be employed. In this technique, a thin piece of skin is harvested from a donor site elsewhere on the body – typically a hairless area like the inner thigh or buttock – and then carefully sutured into the defect created by excising the original scar. The graft essentially replaces the scarred tissue with healthy skin. While this can effectively eliminate the wide or irregular scar, it introduces a new scar at the donor site, and the grafted skin may have a different color and texture than the surrounding skin, potentially appearing slightly paler or more irregular. The graft also requires a vascular supply to be established from the recipient bed, which can take time and may sometimes lead to partial or complete graft loss if this "take" is not successful. Despite these potential drawbacks, skin grafting is a valuable tool for resurfacing large or complex scar defects where direct closure is not feasible.

Another sophisticated surgical technique for scar revision is the **Z-plasty**. This method is particularly useful for scars that are not aligned with the RSTLs, or for scar contractures that are pulling the skin in an undesirable direction.

A Z-plasty involves excising the scar and then making two triangular flaps of skin on either side of the wound. These flaps are then transposed and sut closure, creating a "Z" shape in the wound closure line. This transposition effectively breaks up the straight line of the original scar and allows the surgeon to realign the wound edges in a different direction. By strategically orienting the Z-plasty, the surgeon can reposition the resulting scar to lie along the RSTLs, thereby reducing tension and making it less noticeable. Z-plasties are often employed for scars crossing joints, around the eyes, or on the face where scar orientation is critical for aesthetic outcome. The technique can involve multiple geometric variations of the Z, including the W-plasty, which uses a series of small triangular flaps to break up a scar line.

While effective, Z-plasties can sometimes result in a slightly more complex scar pattern than a simple linear closure, and the effectiveness depends heavily on the surgeon's skill and the specific scar characteristics.

For very extensive scarring, particularly those resulting from severe burns or trauma that have led to significant tissue loss and contractures, **tissue expansion** offers a remarkable solution. This technique involves surgically inserting a balloon-like device, known as a tissue expander, under the skin adjacent to the scar.

Over a period of weeks to months, the expander is gradually inflated with saline through a small port. This slow, controlled stretching causes the surrounding healthy skin to grow and expand. Once the desired amount of skin has been generated, the expander is surgically removed, and the expanded skin is then used to cover the area of the original scar, which is typically excised prior to the flap creation.

Tissue expansion allows for the replacement of scarred tissue with healthy, matching skin of the same colour and texture, and it can be used to reconstruct large areas with minimal donor site morbidity. This method requires multiple surgical procedures and a significant time commitment but can yield excellent results for complex reconstructions.

The journey of surgical scar revision begins long before the scalpel touches the skin. The **pre-operative consultation** is a crucial phase where the patient and surgeon engage in a thorough discussion about the scar, the patient's goals, and the available treatment options. The surgeon will meticulously examine the scar, assessing its age, depth, width, colour, texture, and location. They will consider the patient's skin type, healing history, and any predisposition to forming hypertrophic scars or keloids. Realistic expectations are set: surgical revision aims to improve the scar's appearance and function, but it is important to understand that a new scar will always form. The surgeon will explain the different surgical techniques that might be appropriate, outlining the potential benefits, risks, and limitations of each. This is also the time to discuss any pre-existing medical conditions or medications that could affect the surgery or healing process. Detailed pre-operative instructions, including guidelines on medications to avoid (such as blood thinners) and when to stop eating and drinking before the procedure, will be provided.

The **surgical procedure** itself, regardless of the specific technique chosen, is typically performed under sterile conditions in an operating room or a specialized surgical suite. The type of anaesthesia used will depend on the extent and complexity of the revision, as well as the patient's preference and tolerance.

Minor revisions might be performed under local anaesthesia, where the area is numbed with an injection, allowing the patient to remain awake. For more extensive procedures, or for patients who may experience anxiety, intravenous sedation or general anaesthesia may be employed. The surgeon will meticulously cleanse and prepare the skin around the scar. Using precise instruments, the old scar tissue is carefully excised. Once the defect is created, the surgeon will then proceed with the chosen closure method – direct closure with sutures, placement of a skin graft, creation of Z-plasty flaps, or preparation for tissue expander insertion. The closure will be performed using fine sutures, often with both deep sutures to provide structural support and finer sutures for skin approximation to minimize any marks. The duration of the surgery can vary significantly, from under an hour for a simple excision to several hours for complex reconstructions involving tissue expansion.

Following the surgery, the **post-operative care** is paramount to ensure optimal healing and to minimize the risk of complications. The treated area will typically be covered with a sterile dressing to protect the wound. Patients will receive detailed instructions on how to care for the incision site, including how often to change the dressing, how to keep it clean, and what signs of infection to watch for (such as increased redness, swelling, pain, or pus).

Pain management will be addressed with prescribed pain medication. It is common to experience some degree of swelling, bruising, and discomfort in the treated area for the first few days to weeks, which can be managed with elevation and prescribed medications. Patients will be advised to avoid strenuous activities, heavy lifting, or any actions that could put tension on the healing incision.

Sun protection is critically important, as new scars are highly susceptible to hyperpigmentation when exposed to ultraviolet radiation. The surgeon will schedule follow-up appointments to monitor the healing progress, remove sutures at the appropriate time (usually within 5-10 days, depending on the location), and assess the initial outcome.

The **recovery period** after surgical scar revision is a gradual process. While the initial discomfort and swelling usually subside within a week or two, the scar itself will continue to mature and refine over many months, sometimes up to a year or even longer.

During this maturation phase, the initial redness will gradually fade, and the scar will typically soften and flatten. Early post-operative management often involves the use of silicone sheets or gels, massage, and sometimes topical or intralesional corticosteroid injections to help prevent the scar from becoming raised or hypertrophic. Patients are usually advised to continue protecting the scar from the sun for at least a year.

It is essential for patients to adhere strictly to all post-operative instructions and to attend all scheduled follow-up appointments to ensure the best possible outcome.

It is imperative to reiterate the concept of **realistic expectations**.

Surgical scar revision is a powerful tool for improving the appearance and function of problematic scars, but it does not guarantee the complete disappearance of the scar. The goal is to transform a conspicuous, undesirable scar into one that is less noticeable, better aligned, and less functionally limiting. The resulting scar, while often significantly improved, will still be present.

The success of the revision depends on numerous factors, including the initial scar characteristics, the surgical technique employed, the skill of the surgeon, and the individual's healing response. In some cases, multiple revision procedures may be necessary to achieve the desired aesthetic outcome.

For individuals with a history of keloid formation, there remains a risk of recurrence, and close monitoring and preventative treatments may be required. Ultimately, surgical scar revision is a highly effective option for those seeking to address the most challenging and persistent scar concerns, offering a pathway to a more aesthetically pleasing and functionally restored outcome.

# Chapter Five

## Managing Expectations and Psychological Well-being

The journey of a scar from its inception is a dynamic and prolonged one, marked by distinct phases of maturation. It is crucial to understand that a scar is not a static entity; rather, it is a living tissue that undergoes a profound transformation over time. This evolutionary process, often referred to as scar maturation, is lengthy and can extend anywhere from 12 to 24 months, and in some cases, even longer. Appreciating this timeline is not merely an academic exercise; it is fundamental to managing expectations and fostering psychological well-being throughout the healing process. Rushing interventions or becoming disheartened by initial appearances can lead to unnecessary anxiety and potentially suboptimal outcomes. Instead, embracing patience and understanding the natural course of scar development allows for a more realistic and ultimately more satisfying journey toward scar resolution.

In the initial weeks and months following injury or surgery, the scar typically enters what is often described as the proliferative or inflammatory phase. During this period, the wound is actively healing, characterized by robust cellular activity aimed at repairing the damaged tissue. Clinically, this translates into a scar that may appear red, raised, and sometimes slightly tender or itchy.

The redness is a direct result of increased blood flow to the area as part of the inflammatory response and the formation of new, immature blood vessels. The raised appearance is due to the deposition of collagen, a key protein in scar tissue, which is laid down in a disorganized manner during this active healing phase. This can lead to a scar that is not only elevated above the surrounding skin but may also feel firm to the touch.

Itching is also a common sensation as nerve endings regenerate and the skin's healing mechanisms are at play. For many, this phase can be the most challenging visually and sensationally. The redness can be quite pronounced, and the elevation noticeable, leading some to believe the scar is worse than it will ultimately become. It is precisely during this stage that patience is most critical. The scar is still very much in its developmental infancy, and its appearance at this point is not indicative of its final form. Attempting significant interventions during this hyperactive phase can sometimes disrupt the delicate healing process and may even exacerbate redness or raise the scar further.

As the months progress, typically from around the 3-month mark onward, the scar begins to transition into the remodelling or maturation phase. This is where the real magic of natural scar healing begins to occur, albeit at a slow and steady pace. During this phase, the body continues its work, but the focus shifts from rapid proliferation to organized reconstruction. The haphazardly deposited collagen fibres start to realign themselves, becoming more parallel and organized. This reorganization strengthens the scar tissue and, crucially, leads to a gradual flattening and softening. The increased vascularity that contributed to the initial redness begins to decrease, causing the colour of the scar to fade.

What was once a vibrant red hue will slowly transform into a more muted pink, and eventually, over a much longer period, to a pale, silvery, or white line that closely matches the surrounding skin tone. This process of remodelling can take many months, often extending to a full year or even two years post-injury or surgery. It is this extended duration that underscores the importance of patience. The visible improvements during the maturation phase are often subtle from week to week, but significant when viewed over several months. Patients who monitor their scars daily might not notice incremental changes, but revisiting photographs taken a few months apart will often reveal a dramatic difference in the scar's colour, texture, and elevation.

Understanding these stages is paramount for managing expectations. A patient undergoing scar revision surgery, for example, will have an initial incision that is essentially a "fresh" scar. This new scar will go through the same maturation process as any other wound. Immediately after surgery, it will likely appear as a thin, red line.

It might be slightly raised due to initial inflammation and collagen deposition. Expecting it to look like a mature, almost invisible scar within weeks is unrealistic and sets the stage for disappointment. Instead, the focus immediately post-op should be on meticulous wound care and protection, allowing the initial healing to occur without complications. As the weeks turn into months, the patient should anticipate the gradual changes outlined: fading redness, softening texture, and flattening of the scar. This natural maturation is often the most significant contributor to scar improvement.

The psychological impact of understanding this timeline cannot be overstated.

For individuals who have undergone surgery or experienced an injury, the scar can be a constant reminder of the event, impacting self-esteem and body image. When a scar appears angry and prominent in the early weeks, it can fuel anxiety and distress. However, knowing that this is a temporary phase and that the scar is on a predictable, albeit slow, trajectory toward improvement can provide immense comfort and resilience. This knowledge empowers patients to approach their recovery with a more positive outlook, recognizing that healing is a process, not an instantaneous event. It encourages them to focus on the steps they can take to support healing – such as diligent sun protection, appropriate topical treatments, and following post-operative instructions – rather than fixating on the scar's current appearance.

This understanding also informs the timing of further interventions. While treatments like silicone sheeting, topical scar creams, and massage are often recommended from the early stages of healing, more intensive therapies such as laser treatments or steroid injections are typically reserved for later in the maturation process. Lasers, for instance, are often most effective when targeting the vascularity of a maturing red scar, or when addressing textural irregularities that become more apparent as the scar flattens. Intralesional corticosteroid injections are commonly used to soften and flatten raised, hypertrophic scars, but their effectiveness can be influenced by the scar's maturity. Performing these interventions too early, when the scar is still in its highly inflammatory proliferative phase, may yield less optimal results or even lead to unwanted side effects. Therefore, a healthcare provider will often advise waiting several months for the scar to progress through its initial healing phases before recommending more aggressive treatments.

This phased approach, dictated by the scar's natural maturation timeline, maximizes the chances of success and patient satisfaction.

Consider the example of a surgical scar on the face. Immediately after surgery, it will be a noticeable line. If the patient understands that it will likely be red and somewhat raised for a few months, they can mentally prepare for this phase. They can also focus on diligent sun protection, knowing that UV exposure can darken the scar and make it more prominent during this sensitive period. As the scar begins to fade and soften over the next six to twelve months, the patient will likely feel a sense of relief and accomplishment, seeing the natural improvements unfold. If the scar remains significantly raised or pigmented after a year, then targeted treatments like laser therapy or steroid injections can be considered, with a much higher likelihood of success because the scar is no longer in its volatile early stages.

Similarly, for scars resulting from acne, trauma, or burns, the maturation process follows the same principles. An acne scar that initially appears as a red post-inflammatory lesion will gradually fade over time. A traumatic scar will evolve from a raw, red wound to a more subtle line. A burn scar, which can be particularly prone to hypertrophic development, will still undergo a maturation process, albeit often a more prolonged and challenging one, where flattening and softening occur over many months.

In all these scenarios, early intervention based on impatience can be counterproductive. For instance, aggressively trying to "remove" the redness of a very new scar with intense light therapy might lead to paradoxical worsening or pigmentary changes.

Patience allows the body's own healing mechanisms to do the heavy lifting, and then, for persistent concerns, more targeted interventions can be applied to refine the scar's appearance.

It is also important to differentiate between scar maturation and the healing of surgical incisions or wounds. While the principles of scar maturation apply universally, the initial healing of a surgical wound is about primary closure and preventing infection, followed by the subsequent maturation of the resulting scar. The focus in the immediate post-operative period is on keeping the wound clean, closed, and free from tension. As the wound edges seal and the initial inflammatory response subsides, the scar begins its long journey of remodelling. This distinction helps patients understand that the "healing" of a surgical site involves two distinct, though overlapping, phases: wound healing and scar maturation.

The psychological well-being component is profoundly influenced by this temporal perspective. When patients are equipped with knowledge about the scar maturation timeline, they can navigate the emotional rollercoaster of healing with greater equanimity. They learn to distinguish between temporary inflammatory changes and more permanent textural or colour issues. This foresight can prevent premature despair and foster a sense of control over the healing process. Instead of feeling like a victim of a permanent blemish, they can see themselves as active participants in a long-term improvement plan, with patience as a primary tool. This proactive mindset is invaluable for maintaining motivation and for achieving ultimately higher levels of satisfaction with the scar's final appearance.

In conclusion, the timeline of scar maturation is a testament to the body's remarkable capacity for repair and regeneration. This process, stretching over 12 to 24 months or more, dictates a crucial need for patience in scar management. From the initial redness and elevation to the eventual softening and fading, each stage offers insights into what to expect and when to consider further interventions. By understanding and respecting this natural evolution, individuals can approach their scars with realistic expectations, fostering greater psychological resilience and paving the way for more successful and satisfying long-term outcomes. Patience is not just a virtue in scar management; it is a fundamental component that allows the body's natural healing processes to work their best, often achieving significant improvements without the need for aggressive or premature treatments.

The pursuit of "scar removal" is a common desire, often fueled by media portrayals and a wish for an unblemished appearance. However, as medical professionals, it's our responsibility to ground this aspiration in reality. The truth is, in the vast majority of cases, complete scar removal is not a feasible outcome. Instead, the focus of modern scar management, whether through surgical techniques, topical treatments, or advanced therapies, is unequivocally on **scar improvement**. This means making a scar less conspicuous, less noticeable, and more harmonious with the surrounding skin. Think of it as refining and blending, rather than erasing. The aim is to transform a scar from a prominent feature into a subtle line, or a textural difference that is easily overlooked, rather than achieving a state where the skin appears as if no injury or procedure ever occurred. This distinction is fundamental to establishing a realistic psychological framework for anyone navigating the scar healing journey.

Understanding what "less noticeable" entails requires a look at various scar types and their potential for improvement. For instance, a fine, linear surgical scar, particularly one that has undergone adequate maturation, can often be improved to the point where it is barely visible to the naked eye. This might involve reducing any residual redness, flattening any subtle elevation, and ensuring the colour blends well with the adjacent skin. Treatments like silicone sheeting, topical retinoids, or gentle massage can facilitate this kind of subtle refinement by promoting collagen organization and reducing inflammation.

In such cases, the improvement can be so significant that, under normal viewing conditions, the scar is easily missed. This is a prime example of what successful scar improvement looks like – a harmonious integration of the healed tissue with its surroundings.

However, not all scars are created equal, and their potential for improvement varies. Consider hypertrophic scars – those raised, often red scars that remain confined to the original wound boundaries. While significant improvement is possible, completely flattening them to the level of the surrounding skin can be challenging. Treatments such as corticosteroid injections, silicone gel applications, and sometimes even surgical revision can help to soften, flatten, and reduce the redness of these scars.

The outcome might be a scar that is much less prominent, smoother, and paler, but a complete disappearance of its raised character may not always be achievable.

The residual elevation might still be palpable or subtly visible, representing a significant improvement, but not a total obliteration.

Keloid scars present an even greater challenge. These are scars that grow beyond the original boundaries of the wound, often appearing as thick, rubbery, and sometimes unsightly growths. Keloids are notorious for their tendency to recur even after treatment, and for some individuals, achieving a scar that is truly "less noticeable" can be a long and arduous process with a higher likelihood of recurrence. Treatments like cryotherapy, corticosteroid injections, radiation therapy (in specific cases), and surgical excision with adjunctive therapies are employed. The goal here is often to reduce the size and thickness of the keloid and manage symptoms like itching or pain. While a successful outcome might involve a scar that is considerably smaller and less symptomatic than the original keloid, it is unlikely to become an invisible line. The improved keloid might be flatter and less aggressive, but it will likely remain a visible alteration to the skin.

Acne scars, especially the atrophic types like icepick, boxcar, and rolling scars, also fall into the category of improvement rather than eradication. These scars represent a loss of tissue, creating depressions in the skin. Treatments like chemical peels, microdermabrasion, laser resurfacing, microneedling, and dermal fillers are used to stimulate collagen production, improve skin texture, and fill in the depressions. While these modalities can dramatically improve the overall appearance of the skin, making the scars much less obvious and the complexion smoother, they cannot fully regenerate the lost tissue to pre-acne levels. The outcome is a smoother, more even-toned skin surface with significantly reduced scar visibility, but the underlying textural irregularities may not be entirely eliminated.

The type of injury or procedure plays a crucial role in determining the potential for scar improvement. A clean, precise surgical incision made by a skilled surgeon on an area of skin with good elasticity will typically result in a scar that is far more amenable to improvement than a wide, jagged wound from trauma or a complex scar from a severe burn. For example, a scar from a laparoscopic surgery on the abdomen, often characterized by small puncture marks, can usually be improved to become almost imperceptible with time and appropriate care. In contrast, a large scar from a third-degree burn might involve significant tissue loss, contracture, and altered skin texture and colour, making complete "disappearance" a remote possibility. While interventions can significantly improve function and appearance, the scar will likely remain a noticeable feature, albeit a much less restrictive or disfiguring one.

Furthermore, the age of the scar is a critical factor. As discussed previously, scars mature over time. While early intervention can sometimes be beneficial for managing inflammation and improving texture, attempting to aggressively treat a very new scar might be premature. Conversely, very old scars may have undergone their natural maturation process and might be less responsive to treatments that rely on influencing active healing or inflammation. However, certain treatments, like fractional laser resurfacing, can sometimes rejuvenate older scar tissue and improve its texture and colour, demonstrating that improvement is possible even years after the initial injury. The key is understanding the scar's current state and choosing treatments accordingly, always with the aim of improvement, not eradication.

The patient's inherent skin characteristics also profoundly influence the outcomes of scar treatments. Individuals with darker skin tones (Fitzpatrick types IV-VI) are at a higher risk of post-inflammatory hyperpigmentation (PIH) or hypopigmentation following many scar treatments, particularly those involving inflammation or laser energy. This means that while the scar itself might improve, the surrounding skin could develop darker or lighter patches, which can be a new concern for the patient. Dermatologists and plastic surgeons must carefully select treatments and protocols for these individuals to minimize these risks. For example, gentler resurfacing techniques or depigmenting agents might be prioritized. Similarly, individuals prone to keloid formation may experience recurrence even after seemingly successful scar revision, highlighting the body's individual response to injury and healing.

Adherence to treatment protocols is another non-negotiable factor in achieving realistic outcomes. Many scar improvement strategies require consistent, long-term application. For example, regular application of silicone gel or sheets for several months, diligent sun protection, and performing prescribed scar massage are crucial for optimizing the results of surgical scars. Similarly, a course of chemical peels or laser treatments requires multiple sessions and diligent post-treatment care, including strict sun avoidance and the use of prescribed topical agents. Patients who are diligent in following these instructions are far more likely to achieve the best possible improvement. Conversely, inconsistent application or neglecting post-treatment care can significantly diminish the effectiveness of even the most advanced interventions, leading to less favourable results and potential frustration.

It is also essential to manage expectations regarding the *degree* of improvement.

While a scar might be improved by 50%, 75%, or even 90%, it is rarely improved by 100%. This gradual reduction in noticeability is the tangible goal. For example, a raised, red scar might be softened and faded to a pale, flat line. This is a significant improvement, but it is still a scar. If the expectation was for the skin to return to its pristine, unscarred state, then this excellent outcome might be perceived as a failure. Therefore, open and honest communication between the patient and the healthcare provider about the *potential* for improvement, rather than the *certainty* of disappearance, is paramount. This involves discussing what the scar looks like now, what it is likely to look like after treatment, and what limitations exist for that specific scar type and individual.

Consider the psychological impact of this realistic outlook. When patients understand that the goal is improvement, they are less likely to experience profound disappointment if a scar doesn't vanish completely. Instead, they can celebrate the progress made and appreciate the enhanced appearance and function. This realistic framing can foster greater satisfaction with the treatment journey and the final result, even if the scar remains detectable to a trained eye.

It shifts the focus from an unattainable ideal to achievable enhancements, empowering patients to feel more in control and less disheartened by perceived imperfections. This nuanced understanding is crucial for maintaining motivation throughout the often lengthy process of scar management.

In summary, the concept of "scar removal" is largely a misnomer in the realm of medical and cosmetic treatments.

The realistic goal and achievable outcome for virtually all scars is **improvement**, aiming to make them less noticeable, less conspicuous, and more harmonious with the surrounding skin. The degree of improvement varies significantly based on scar type, age, location, patient skin characteristics, and adherence to treatment. By embracing this reality, patients can embark on their scar management journey with grounded expectations, appreciating the significant enhancements that can be achieved through various therapeutic modalities, and fostering a more positive and ultimately more satisfying experience.

The presence of a scar, regardless of its size or location, can extend far beyond the physical realm, deeply influencing an individual's psychological landscape. This impact is not always immediate; sometimes it is a slow, creeping realization that the healed wound has become a permanent alteration, a visible reminder of a past event, be it an accident, surgery, or a medical condition. For many, this can trigger a cascade of complex emotional responses that shape their self-perception and their engagement with the world around them. It is vital to acknowledge and validate these feelings, recognizing that the emotional toll of scarring is a significant aspect of the healing process, one that deserves as much attention as the physical management of the scar itself.

Commonly, individuals living with scars may experience a profound sense of loss. This loss is not just of the pristine skin that existed before, but often a loss of a perceived sense of normalcy, of an unblemished self-image that may have been integral to their identity. This can manifest as a diminished self-esteem. When one looks in the mirror and sees a scar, it can trigger a critical internal dialogue, focusing on what is perceived as imperfection.

This persistent self-scrutiny can erode confidence, making individuals feel self-conscious and less assured in social situations or even in intimate relationships. The scar can become the focal point of their self-perception, overshadowing other qualities and achievements.

Anxiety is another pervasive emotional response. This anxiety can be multifaceted. It might be a fear of judgment from others – the worry that people will stare, comment, or make assumptions based on the scar. This fear can lead to a constant state of vigilance, where social interactions are approached with apprehension. For some, the anxiety is tied to the origin of the scar; if it resulted from a traumatic event, the scar can serve as a constant, unconscious trigger, bringing back memories and the associated distress. This can lead to avoidance behaviours, where individuals actively steer clear of situations that might draw attention to their scar or trigger distressing memories.

Depression can also be a significant consequence of living with scarring. When the emotional burden of self-consciousness, anxiety, and a diminished sense of self becomes overwhelming, it can lead to a feeling of hopelessness and a loss of interest in activities that once brought joy. The persistent feeling of being different, of not fitting in with societal ideals of beauty or perfection, can be profoundly isolating. This isolation, whether self-imposed due to fear of judgment or a natural consequence of withdrawal, can exacerbate feelings of sadness and despair. The feeling of being "marked" can contribute to a sense of being fundamentally flawed, which can be a heavy weight to carry.

Social withdrawal is a frequent coping mechanism, albeit an unhealthy one, for individuals struggling with the psychological impact of scarring.

To avoid potential scrutiny, embarrassment, or uncomfortable questions, some may choose to limit their social interactions. This can mean declining invitations to social events, avoiding activities that involve revealing clothing (like swimming or beach outings), or even limiting their professional opportunities if they feel the scar could negatively impact their career prospects. This withdrawal, while intended to protect them from perceived harm, ultimately leads to greater isolation and can deepen the feelings of depression and low self-esteem, creating a cyclical pattern of emotional distress.

It is crucial to emphasize that these emotional responses are not signs of weakness or oversensitivity. They are, in fact, entirely normal and understandable reactions to living with a visible alteration of one's body. Our society often places a high value on physical appearance, and the media frequently promotes an ideal of flawless skin. When an individual bears a scar, they are, in a sense, deviating from this idealized norm. This deviation can lead to internal and external pressures that are difficult to navigate. Recognizing that many others share these experiences can be incredibly validating. Understanding that feeling anxious, sad, or self-conscious is a common human response to scarring helps to destigmatize these emotions and allows individuals to begin the process of healing not just their skin, but their emotional well-being too.

The journey towards psychological well-being when living with scars involves developing effective coping mechanisms and actively seeking support. One powerful strategy is the practice of mindfulness. Mindfulness involves paying attention to the present moment without judgment. For someone with a scar, this can mean acknowledging the scar's presence without immediately attaching negative emotions to it.

It's about observing the sensation of the skin, the awareness of its texture, or even the visual appearance, with a sense of detached curiosity rather than harsh criticism. Regular mindfulness meditation, deep breathing exercises, or simply taking a few moments to focus on one's breath can help to ground individuals, interrupt cycles of anxious thoughts, and create a greater sense of calm and acceptance. By practicing mindfulness, individuals can learn to observe their thoughts and feelings about their scar without being consumed by them, gradually reducing their power.

Positive self-talk is another vital tool. This involves consciously challenging negative or critical thoughts about oneself and replacing them with more balanced, compassionate, and realistic affirmations. Instead of thinking, "This scar makes me ugly," one might reframe it as, "This scar is a part of my story. It doesn't define my worth or my beauty." This requires practice and intentional effort. It might involve writing down positive affirmations, repeating them daily, or actively noticing and countering negative self-commentary as it arises. The goal is not to deny the existence of the scar or the feelings associated with it, but to shift the internal narrative from one of criticism and self-rejection to one of self-compassion and acceptance. Celebrating small victories, such as wearing a certain outfit without excessive worry or engaging in a social activity despite initial apprehension, can also reinforce positive self-perception.

Seeking support, whether from friends, family, or professional resources, is paramount. Sharing one's feelings with trusted individuals can alleviate feelings of isolation and provide emotional validation. Sometimes, simply articulating one's struggles aloud can be a cathartic experience.

It is important to surround oneself with people who are understanding and supportive, individuals who see beyond the scar and appreciate the person as a whole. These relationships can provide a sense of belonging and reinforce the individual's value.

For those whose psychological distress is more profound or persistent, seeking professional help from a therapist or counsellor is highly recommended. Therapists specializing in body image issues, trauma, or anxiety can provide tailored strategies and support. Cognitive Behavioural Therapy (CBT), for instance, is highly effective in identifying and modifying negative thought patterns and behaviours associated with self-consciousness and anxiety. Eye Movement Desensitization and Reprocessing (EMDR) therapy can be particularly helpful if the scar is linked to a traumatic event, helping to process and neutralize the associated distress.

Support groups, both online and in-person, specifically for individuals with scars, can offer a unique sense of community and shared understanding. Hearing from others who have navigated similar challenges can provide invaluable insights, practical advice, and a powerful reminder that one is not alone.

It's also important to approach scar management treatments with a holistic perspective. While the physical treatments aim to improve the scar's appearance, they should also be viewed as part of a broader journey of self-care. Engaging in treatments can be an act of empowerment, a way of taking control and actively working towards feeling better.

However, it is crucial to maintain realistic expectations about the outcomes of these treatments, as discussed previously.

When treatments are viewed as tools for improvement rather than complete eradication, and when they are coupled with robust psychological coping strategies, the overall impact on well-being is significantly enhanced.

Ultimately, living with a scar is about integration, not erasure. It is about weaving the scar into the fabric of one's life story, recognizing it as a testament to resilience and survival, rather than a mark of imperfection. By understanding the psychological impact of scarring, validating the associated emotions, and actively employing coping strategies and seeking support, individuals can navigate this journey with greater strength, confidence, and a profound sense of self-acceptance. Prioritizing mental and emotional well-being is not a secondary concern; it is an integral component of comprehensive scar management, leading to a more fulfilling and empowered life.

The journey of healing from a scar is multifaceted, extending beyond the physical repair of tissue to encompass the profound psychological and emotional landscape of the individual. While self-care strategies, positive affirmations, and the support of loved ones can be invaluable in navigating the complexities of living with a visible mark, there are times when professional intervention becomes not just beneficial, but essential. Recognizing when to seek external help and understanding how to access it are critical steps in ensuring comprehensive well-being.

The decision to seek professional support is often precipitated by the persistence or exacerbation of emotional distress. If feelings of low mood, anxiety, or self-consciousness surrounding a scar begin to interfere significantly with daily life, it may be an indication that professional guidance is warranted.

This interference can manifest in various ways: a pervasive sense of sadness that doesn't lift, constant worry about how others perceive the scar, or an increasing tendency to avoid social situations, activities, or even certain clothing choices that might draw attention to the area.

When these emotional responses become chronic, debilitating, or lead to a significant decline in quality of life, it's a clear signal that the individual could benefit from the expertise of a mental health professional.

Consider, for instance, a situation where an individual who once enjoyed swimming or participating in sports now consistently declines invitations due to embarrassment about a scar on their leg.

This avoidance, if sustained, can lead to a gradual erosion of social connections and a loss of activities that were once a source of joy and physical health.

Similarly, if a scar impacts an individual's confidence in their professional life, leading them to shy away from presentations or networking opportunities, this can have tangible career consequences.

These are not merely minor inconveniences; they are significant disruptions that suggest the emotional impact of the scar is overshadowing other aspects of the individual's life.

Another critical indicator for seeking help is the presence of symptoms suggestive of anxiety disorders or depression.

Persistent irritability, changes in sleep patterns (insomnia or excessive sleeping), alterations in appetite, a loss of interest in previously enjoyed activities, or feelings of hopelessness can all be signs that a more serious mood disorder may be developing or worsening.

If the scar is associated with a traumatic event – such as an accident, assault, or a difficult medical procedure – and triggers intrusive thoughts, flashbacks, or nightmares, this could indicate Post-Traumatic Stress Disorder (PTSD) or a related trauma response. In such cases, specialized therapeutic interventions are crucial.

The role of a therapist or counsellor is to provide a safe, non-judgmental space where individuals can explore their feelings and experiences related to their scar. These professionals are trained to identify and address the underlying psychological mechanisms that contribute to distress. They can offer a range of therapeutic modalities tailored to the individual's specific needs. Cognitive Behavioural Therapy (CBT), for example, is highly effective in helping individuals challenge and reframe negative thought patterns associated with their scar. For instance, if someone constantly thinks, "Everyone is staring at my scar," CBT can help them identify the evidence for this thought, examine alternative explanations, and develop more balanced and realistic perspectives. The therapist works collaboratively with the patient to develop coping strategies for managing anxious thoughts and to gradually reintroduce them to situations they have been avoiding.

For scars resulting from trauma, therapies like Eye Movement Desensitization and Reprocessing (EMDR) can be particularly beneficial. EMDR is designed to help the brain process traumatic memories that have become "stuck," reducing the emotional intensity associated with them. By guiding the individual through specific bilateral stimulation (often eye movements) while recalling distressing memories and associated sensations, EMDR can help to desensitize these memories, making them less intrusive and less likely to trigger distress.

This can be transformative for individuals who feel haunted by the event that caused their scar.

Beyond individual therapy, support groups can offer a unique and powerful form of assistance. These groups bring together individuals who share similar experiences, creating a sense of community and shared understanding that is often difficult to find elsewhere. In a scar support group, members can openly discuss their feelings, fears, and challenges without fear of judgment or misunderstanding. They can share practical tips for managing the physical and emotional aspects of scarring, offer encouragement, and provide invaluable peer support. Hearing from others who have successfully navigated similar emotional terrain can be incredibly empowering and can combat the sense of isolation that often accompanies visible differences. Support groups can be found both online and in person, catering to a wide range of scar types and causes.

When considering professional help, it's important to find a mental health professional who has experience with issues related to body image, self-esteem, anxiety, depression, or trauma. Many therapists specialize in these areas. Resources for finding such professionals include recommendations from your primary care physician or dermatologist, online directories of licensed therapists (such as Psychology Today's therapist finder), and reputable mental health organizations. When you first connect with a potential therapist, it's appropriate to ask about their experience with individuals dealing with scarring or body image concerns. Don't hesitate to schedule introductory consultations with a few different therapists to find someone with whom you feel a strong connection and trust. The therapeutic relationship is a cornerstone of successful treatment.

The process of finding support should be viewed as an active and empowering step in the healing journey. It is not a sign of weakness, but rather a testament to one's commitment to overall well-being. Just as one would seek medical attention for a persistent physical ailment, seeking psychological support for emotional distress is a proactive and responsible approach to health. By understanding the signs that professional help might be beneficial, knowing the types of support available, and actively seeking out qualified professionals and groups, individuals can effectively address the psychological impact of scarring, leading to greater resilience, acceptance, and a richer, more fulfilling life. This proactive engagement with one's mental health complements and enhances the physical treatments aimed at scar improvement, creating a holistic path towards healing and self-empowerment.

The journey toward accepting and embracing your skin, with or without scars, is a deeply personal and often transformative process. While professional support and therapeutic interventions discussed previously can be invaluable in navigating the emotional complexities of scarring, there's a profound power in cultivating internal resilience and self-assurance.

This chapter delves into strategies for building confidence, not by erasing what makes you unique, but by celebrating it. It's about shifting the narrative from one of perceived imperfection to one of inherent worth and strength.

At the heart of this shift is the practice of self-compassion. Often, we are our own harshest critics, holding ourselves to impossibly high standards and dwelling on perceived flaws. When it comes to scars, this internal dialogue can be particularly relentless.

Self-compassion, however, invites us to treat ourselves with the same kindness, understanding, and acceptance we would offer a dear friend. It means acknowledging that everyone experiences hardship, everyone bears marks, visible or invisible, and that these experiences are part of the human condition. Instead of berating yourself for a scar, or for the feelings it evokes, practice offering yourself a gentler perspective. This might involve saying to yourself, "This is difficult, and it's okay to feel this way. My scar is a part of my story, and it doesn't diminish my value." It's about recognizing your own pain without judgment and offering yourself comfort and understanding. This practice doesn't negate the desire for improvement or healing, but it ensures that the process is rooted in self-love, not self-loathing.

Cultivating a strong sense of self-esteem extends beyond passive acceptance; it involves actively engaging with your strengths and valuing your unique qualities. Scars, while often the focus of concern, are only one facet of who you are. Take time to identify and appreciate your many other attributes: your intelligence, your creativity, your kindness, your resilience, your sense of humor, your skills, your passions, your relationships. Make a conscious effort to acknowledge these aspects of yourself daily. Perhaps keeping a journal where you list things you like about yourself, or accomplishments you're proud of, can be a powerful tool. When you feel a wave of insecurity related to a scar, consciously bring your attention to these other strengths. Remind yourself of all the wonderful things that make you, *you*. This isn't about denial; it's about a balanced perspective, ensuring that your self-worth isn't solely tied to your physical appearance.

Engaging in activities that genuinely bring you joy and a sense of accomplishment can also be a significant confidence booster. These are activities where you can focus on your abilities and feel competent and fulfilled. Whether it's mastering a new recipe, learning a musical instrument, excelling at a sport, creating art, volunteering your time, or achieving a professional milestone, these experiences reinforce your capabilities and build a sense of agency. The endorphins released through physical activity, the satisfaction of learning a new skill, or the sense of purpose derived from helping others can all contribute to a more positive self-image. It's about actively creating experiences that build you up, proving to yourself, time and again, that you are capable and valuable, irrespective of any visible marks.

Positive affirmations can serve as powerful anchors in this process of rebuilding confidence. These are short, positive statements that, when repeated regularly, can help to reprogram negative thought patterns and foster a more optimistic outlook. The key to effective affirmations is to make them believable to you and to focus on them with sincerity. Instead of generic statements, tailor them to your specific needs. For example, if you struggle with feeling self-conscious about a scar on your face, an affirmation like, "My face tells a story, and it is beautiful," or "I am confident and radiant," can be more impactful than a general statement about beauty. Repeat these affirmations aloud or in your mind during moments of self-doubt, while looking in the mirror, or as part of your morning routine. Over time, consistent repetition can help to shift your internal dialogue towards more positive and empowering beliefs. It's not about forcing yourself to believe something that feels untrue, but about gently guiding your mind towards a more self-accepting perspective.

The digital age has also opened up avenues to connect with communities that champion body positivity and self-acceptance. These online spaces can provide a sense of belonging and validation, offering a counter-narrative to the often unrealistic beauty standards perpetuated in mainstream media. Engaging with body-positive advocates, following social media accounts that celebrate diverse body types, and participating in online forums where individuals share their journeys of self-love can be incredibly inspiring.

Witnessing others embrace their scars, their stretch marks, their body shapes, and their unique features can normalize your own experience and encourage you to do the same. These communities often provide practical tips, share empowering stories, and offer a supportive network where you can feel seen and understood. Remember, you are not alone in your journey, and connecting with others who are on a similar path can be profoundly validating.

Self-care routines are not just about pampering; they are fundamental acts of self-respect and self-preservation. Establishing consistent self-care practices can significantly contribute to your overall sense of well-being and confidence. This can encompass a wide range of activities, from ensuring adequate sleep and maintaining a balanced diet to engaging in mindful movement and setting healthy boundaries. Consider incorporating activities that nurture your physical and emotional health.

This might include a regular skincare routine that makes you feel good about your skin, even with its marks. It could be gentle exercise that strengthens your body and clears your mind, or time spent in nature, which has been shown to reduce stress and improve mood.

Prioritizing these practices signals to yourself that your well-being is a priority, which in turn bolsters your self-esteem. When you feel physically well and cared for, it becomes easier to project that confidence outwardly.

Moreover, learning to manage your internal dialogue about your scar is a skill that can be honed. When you notice critical thoughts arising, pause and gently question them. Are these thoughts truly accurate, or are they fuelled by insecurity or past negative experiences? Are there alternative, more compassionate interpretations? For example, if you catch yourself thinking, "This scar makes me look so ugly," try reframing it to, "This scar is a reminder of a time I overcame a challenge. It is part of my history." This process of cognitive reframing, often honed with the help of a therapist, is about actively choosing to challenge and change the way you think about yourself and your appearance. It requires practice and patience, but the rewards in terms of increased self-acceptance and confidence are immense.

The concept of viewing your scar as a part of your unique life story is a powerful one.

Scars are not merely blemishes; they are often physical manifestations of experiences, resilience, and survival.

They tell a story of where you've been, what you've endured, and how you've healed.

Instead of viewing them as flaws that detract from your narrative, consider them as chapters that add depth and character to your life's book.

This perspective shift can transform how you feel about your appearance.

It encourages you to see your scar not as something to be hidden or ashamed of, but as a testament to your strength and your journey.

When you embrace this idea, you empower yourself by owning your story, and in doing so, you reclaim your narrative from any potential shame or negativity.

This journey towards building confidence and embracing your skin is an ongoing process, not a destination with a fixed endpoint.

There will be days when you feel more confident and days when insecurity creeps back in. The goal isn't to achieve a constant state of unshakeable self-assurance, but to develop the tools and mindset to navigate these fluctuations with grace and self-compassion.

It's about building a resilient inner foundation that can withstand the inevitable ups and downs. By consistently practicing self-compassion, focusing on your strengths, engaging in fulfilling activities, utilizing positive affirmations, connecting with supportive communities, prioritizing self-care, and reframing your internal dialogue, you can cultivate a deep and lasting sense of self-acceptance and confidence.

Your skin, with all its unique markings, is a canvas that tells the story of your life, and learning to love that story is perhaps the most beautiful transformation of all.

# Chapter Six

## A Personalized Scar Management Plan

Understanding the unique characteristics of your scar is the foundational step in crafting an effective management plan. Before consulting with a medical professional or exploring various treatment options, a thorough self-assessment will empower you with knowledge and clarity, allowing for more informed discussions and realistic expectations. This isn't about self-diagnosis, but rather about becoming an active participant in your own care, armed with a comprehensive understanding of your individual situation. Think of this as gathering the essential data points that will guide the development of a tailored strategy.

To begin this process, let's systematically consider the various attributes of your scar. This structured approach will help ensure that no detail is overlooked. We can break this down into several key areas:

**1. Scar Type:**

The first and perhaps most crucial aspect is identifying the type of scar you have. Different scar types respond differently to treatments, and understanding this classification is paramount.

**Atrophic Scars:** These scars are characterized by a depression or indentation in the skin. They occur when the body doesn't produce enough collagen during the healing process.

**Boxcar Scars:** These are broad depressions with sharply defined edges, often resembling the shape of a boxcar. They are common after acne or chickenpox.

**Ice Pick Scars:** These are narrow, deep-pitted scars that extend into the dermis, giving the skin a pitted appearance like it's been pricked with an ice pick. They are also frequently associated with acne.

**Rolling Scars:** These scars create an uneven, undulating texture on the skin's surface, with sloping edges. They are often caused by the fibrous bands that form under the skin, tethering the epidermis down.

**Hypertrophic Scars:** These scars are raised, red, and sometimes thickened. They develop when the body produces an overabundance of collagen during healing, but the scar remains confined within the original boundaries of the wound. They can improve over time, softening and flattening, but may take months or even years.

**Keloid Scars:** Similar to hypertrophic scars, keloids are raised and often red or purplish.

However, keloids grow beyond the original boundaries of the wound and can continue to expand over time. They are more common in individuals with darker skin tones and can be itchy or painful. Keloids are often more challenging to treat and have a higher rate of recurrence.

**Stretched Scars:** These scars appear as thin, often hypopigmented or

hyperpigmented lines, resulting from skin stretching due to rapid growth (like during puberty or pregnancy) or significant weight fluctuations.

They are commonly seen after surgery where the skin was under tension.

**Contracture Scars:** These scars are often the result of burns or deep wounds. They are characterized by tight, inelastic skin that can restrict movement, particularly around joints, fingers, or the eyelids. The underlying tissue may also be affected.

Take a close look at your scar. Does it sit flat with the surrounding skin, form a depression, or rise above it? Does it appear to have grown beyond the original injury site? Consulting visual aids or discussing these categories with a healthcare provider can be very helpful in accurate identification.

**2. Scar Age and Healing Stage:**

The age of your scar significantly influences its appearance and how it will respond to treatment.

**New Scars (0-6 months):** These are still in the active healing phase. They are typically red, raised (in the case of hypertrophic or keloid scars), and may be sensitive. Treatments during this phase are often focused on preventing excessive collagen formation, reducing redness, and promoting a flatter, less noticeable scar.

Interventions might include silicone sheeting, pressure dressings, topical agents like corticosteroid creams, or intralesional injections.

**Mature Scars (6 months+):** These scars have completed their active remodelling phase. They may still be red, but will typically flatten over time. Hypertrophic scars may have softened. Mature atrophic scars are more established depressions. Treatments for mature scars often focus on improving texture, colour, and contour. This could involve laser therapies, microneedling, fillers, chemical peels, or surgical revision, depending on the scar type and desired outcome.

Consider when your scar formed. Was it from a recent surgery, an old injury, or a chronic condition like acne? This timeline is crucial for determining appropriate interventions.

**3. Scar Location:**

The location of your scar on the body can impact its visibility, your functional concerns, and the types of treatments that are feasible.

**Face and Neck:** Scars in these highly visible areas often carry a greater emotional and psychological impact. Treatments might prioritize aesthetic outcomes, and the thin skin in these regions can influence the choice of procedures.

**Joints and Areas of Movement:** Scars over joints (like knees, elbows) or in areas requiring significant flexibility (like hands, wrists) can be prone to stretching and may impair function, especially if they are contracture scars. Addressing functional limitations might be a primary goal here.

**Trunk and Limbs:** Scars on these areas can vary in visibility depending on clothing. While aesthetic concerns are still relevant, functional aspects might be less critical unless the scar is very large or in a high-friction zone.

**Scalp and Hair-Bearing Areas:** Scars in these regions may result in permanent hair loss. Treatments might focus on camouflaging the scar or considering procedures that can stimulate hair regrowth if possible.

Where is your scar situated? Does its location make you feel self-conscious? Does it affect your ability to move or perform certain activities?

**4. Scar Texture and Contour:**

This refers to the physical feel and shape of the scar.

**Flat and Smooth:** Some scars may be relatively flat but still noticeable due to color differences.

**Raised and Firm:** Characteristic of hypertrophic and keloid scars, these have a palpable elevation.

**Indented or Pitted:** Typical of atrophic scars, these create depressions in the skin's surface.

**Wavy or Irregular:** Rolling scars and some other types can create a non-uniform surface.

**Tight or Contracted:** Contracture scars often feel taut and inflexible.

Gently run your finger over the scar.

How does it feel compared to the surrounding skin?

Is it smooth, rough, bumpy, or tight?

**Scar Colour:**

The colour of a scar can provide clues about its maturity and healing status.

**Red or Pink:** Newer scars, or actively inflamed hypertrophic/keloid scars, often appear red or pink due to increased blood flow to the area.

**Brown or Hyperpigmented:** As scars mature, they can sometimes darken, especially in individuals with darker skin tones.

This is due to an increase in melanin production.

**White or Hypopigmented:** Mature scars, especially those that have undergone significant remodelling or have lost pigment cells, can appear lighter than the surrounding skin.

Observe the colour of your scar.

Is it significantly different from your natural skin tone?

Has its colour changed over time?

**Associated Symptoms:**

Beyond the visual and tactile characteristics, scars can sometimes cause physical discomfort.

**Itching (Pruritus):** This is a very common symptom, particularly with newer or hypertrophic scars. It can be intensely bothersome and interfere with sleep and daily activities.

**Pain or Tenderness:** Some scars, especially those that are deeper, more inflamed, or located over nerves, can be painful or tender to the touch.

**Numbness:** In some cases, nerve damage during the initial injury or surgery can lead to areas of numbness within or around the scar.

**Stiffness or Limited Range of Motion:** As mentioned with contracture scars, tightness can lead to functional limitations.

Do you experience any itching, burning, pain, or numbness associated with your scar?

Is movement restricted in any way?

Once you have carefully considered these aspects of your scar, the next critical step is to articulate your personal goals for scar management. Your objectives will significantly shape the treatment strategy and will be a key point of discussion with your healthcare provider. Reflect on what you hope to achieve.

**Defining Your Personal Goals:**

**Improve Aesthetic Appearance:** For many, the primary goal is to make the scar less noticeable. This could mean reducing redness, flattening a raised scar, filling in an indentation, minimizing discoloration, or improving overall smoothness and texture.

This goal is particularly common for scars on visible areas like the face, hands, or arms.

**Reduce Discomfort:** If your scar is itchy, painful, or causes a burning sensation, alleviating this discomfort is a paramount goal. Addressing these symptoms can significantly improve your quality of life.

**Regain Full Function:** For contracture scars or those located near joints, the aim might be to restore a normal range of motion and eliminate any restriction in movement. This is crucial for maintaining independence and performing daily activities.

**Prevent Scar Progression:** For newer hypertrophic or keloid scars, a key goal might be to intervene early to prevent them from becoming larger, thicker, or more problematic.

**Increase Confidence and Self-Esteem:** While this is often an overarching outcome of other goals, it's worth stating explicitly. Many individuals seek scar management to feel more comfortable and confident in their own skin, to reduce self-consciousness, and to improve their body image.

**Reduce Scar Irritation:** Some scars can be prone to irritation from friction (e.g., clothing, shaving). Managing this might be a specific objective.

When considering your goals, be as specific as possible. Instead of simply saying "make it look better," try to pinpoint what "better" means to you.

Do you want it to blend in more with your skin tone?

Do you want the raised texture to be less prominent?

Do you want the indentation to be smoother?

Think about the impact your scar has on your daily life and your emotional well-being. Are there specific situations where you feel particularly self-conscious about it? Are there activities you avoid because of your scar?

It is also important to approach your goals with a degree of realism. While significant improvements are often possible, complete scar removal is rarely achievable.

Medical professionals aim to optimize the appearance and sensation of a scar, but a scar is, by definition, a permanent mark. Setting realistic expectations from the outset will help ensure you are satisfied with the outcomes of your treatment plan.

Discussing your aspirations openly with your doctor will help them guide you toward treatments that are most likely to achieve your desired results. They can also help you understand what is realistically achievable for your specific scar type and location.

By dedicating time to this thorough self-assessment—evaluating the type, age, location, texture, colour, and any associated symptoms of your scar, and then clearly defining your personal goals—you are equipping yourself with the knowledge and focus needed to embark on a successful scar management journey.

This proactive approach is the cornerstone of a personalized plan, ensuring that the strategies employed are not only medically sound but also perfectly aligned with your individual needs and aspirations.

This detailed understanding forms the bedrock upon which informed decisions about treatment options will be built.

The journey toward effective scar management is rarely a solitary one.

While a thorough self-assessment of your scar's characteristics and a clear articulation of your personal goals are invaluable starting points, they serve as the foundation for a much more critical phase: consulting with qualified healthcare professionals.

This is where personalized medical expertise transforms your understanding and aspirations into a tangible treatment plan.

Navigating this consultation process with confidence and clarity can significantly influence the success and safety of your scar management journey.

The two primary specialists you will likely encounter are dermatologists and plastic surgeons, each bringing a unique and complementary set of skills to the table.

Understanding their roles, what to expect during your visit, and how to best prepare will empower you to maximize the benefit of their professional guidance.

Dermatologists are physicians who specialize in the diagnosis and treatment of conditions affecting the skin, hair, and nails.

Their expertise is crucial for understanding the intricate biological processes involved in scar formation and healing.

A dermatologist can accurately diagnose the specific type of scar you have, differentiating between atrophic, hypertrophic, keloid, and other scar variations based on their visual characteristics, your medical history, and sometimes even through a skin biopsy if the diagnosis is uncertain.

They are adept at managing the inflammatory aspects of scar tissue, which is particularly important for newer scars or those exhibiting signs of active growth, redness, or itching.

Their armamentarium includes a wide array of topical treatments, injectable therapies, light-based treatments (like lasers and photodynamic therapy), and superficial procedures like chemical peels and microneedling.

For instance, a dermatologist might prescribe silicone-based gels or sheets to help flatten and soften hypertrophic scars or keloids, or administer intralesional corticosteroid injections to reduce inflammation and thickness in raised scars. They are also skilled in managing the pigmentation issues that can accompany scarring, such as post-inflammatory hyperpigmentation or hypopigmentation, using targeted treatments.

Furthermore, dermatologists are often the first line of defence in managing scars resulting from dermatological conditions like acne or eczema, and they possess a deep understanding of how underlying skin health influences scar outcomes. Their approach is often rooted in the physiology of the skin and the management of its cellular responses to injury and healing.

Plastic surgeons, on the other hand, are surgeons who specialize in the restoration, reconstruction, or alteration of the human body. While they are also highly skilled in dermatology and wound healing, their expertise often extends to more invasive and reconstructive techniques. Plastic surgeons are adept at addressing scars that cause functional impairment, such as contracture scars that restrict movement, or those that are significantly disfiguring and require surgical revision. They have the surgical skills to excise problematic scars and meticulously close the wound in a way that aims to create a less noticeable, more aesthetically pleasing scar.

This might involve techniques like scar revision surgery, Z-plasty, or skin grafting, particularly for larger or more complex scars, such as those resulting from significant trauma or burns. Beyond surgical correction, plastic surgeons also utilize many of the non-surgical modalities employed by dermatologists, including laser treatments and injectables, often in conjunction with surgical plans. Their perspective is frequently focused on the three-dimensional aspects of scar correction, considering how the scar impacts the overall contour and structure of the surrounding tissues, and how to best achieve a harmonious aesthetic outcome. For scars that significantly affect appearance or function, a plastic surgeon's expertise in surgical reconstruction and aesthetic principles is invaluable.

The synergy between dermatology and plastic surgery is often where the most comprehensive and effective scar management plans are developed. In many cases, a patient may be referred between these specialties, or a team approach involving both might be recommended.

For example, a dermatologist might manage the inflammatory aspects and pigmentation of a scar, while a plastic surgeon might address its texture, contour, and functional limitations through surgical revision. The choice of specialist often depends on the primary concern related to the scar. If the main issue is redness, itching, or minor textural irregularities, a dermatologist might be the initial point of contact.

If the scar is significantly raised, widely spread, causing functional problems, or deeply indented and requiring significant reconstruction, a plastic surgeon may be the more appropriate starting point.

However, it is not uncommon for either specialist to recommend consultation with the other if it falls outside their immediate scope or if a combined approach is deemed most beneficial.

When preparing for your consultation, remember that this is a collaborative process. The more information you can provide, and the more prepared you are with your questions, the more productive the visit will be. Begin by gathering all relevant medical history pertaining to the scar. This includes the cause of the scar (e.g., surgery, injury, acne, burn), the approximate date of the injury or procedure, and any previous treatments you have undergone, along with their outcomes. If you have photos of the scar from different stages of its development, these can be incredibly helpful for the provider to understand its evolution. Be ready to discuss your medical history, including any allergies, current medications (especially those that affect healing or blood clotting, like blood thinners or certain supplements), and any underlying medical conditions (such as diabetes, autoimmune diseases, or a history of poor wound healing).

If you have a predisposition to keloid scarring or hypertrophic scars, or if there is a family history of such, it is crucial to disclose this information.

During the consultation, the healthcare professional will conduct a thorough examination of your scar and the surrounding skin. They will assess its type, size, location, depth, colour, and texture, as well as any functional limitations or symptoms it causes. They will likely ask you detailed questions about your personal goals for scar management. This is where your self-assessment from the previous steps becomes invaluable.

Be prepared to clearly articulate what you hope to achieve: improved aesthetics, reduced discomfort, restored function, or a combination of these. Be specific. Instead of saying "I want it to look better," explain what "better" means to you. For instance, "I want the redness to be gone," or "I want the indentation to be less noticeable," or "I want to be able to fully extend my finger without feeling tightness."

The provider will then discuss the various treatment options available, explaining the potential benefits, risks, and expected outcomes of each. They will consider your scar's specific characteristics, your medical history, your lifestyle, and your personal goals when making recommendations. Treatment options can range widely, from non-invasive topical therapies and silicone sheeting to minimally invasive procedures like corticosteroid injections, laser treatments, chemical peels, and microneedling, to more involved surgical interventions like scar revision or tissue grafting. They will explain the number of sessions typically required for procedures like laser therapy or microneedling, the estimated recovery time, and the potential for side effects or complications. It is important to understand that not all scars can be completely erased, and some treatments may offer improvement rather than complete elimination. Setting realistic expectations is paramount, and your provider will help you understand what is realistically achievable for your specific situation.

Don't hesitate to ask questions. This is your opportunity to gain a comprehensive understanding of your scar and the proposed treatment plan. Some essential questions to consider asking include:

"Based on your assessment, what type of scar do you believe this is?"

"What are the most effective treatment options for my specific scar type and location?"

"What are the potential benefits and risks associated with each recommended treatment?"

"How many treatment sessions will likely be needed, and what is the expected timeline for results?"

"What is the estimated cost of the treatment plan?" (It's important to clarify whether insurance covers any portion of scar treatment, as this often depends on medical necessity versus cosmetic preference).

"What can I expect in terms of discomfort during and after the treatment?"

"What is the expected downtime or recovery period?"

"Are there any home care instructions I should follow?"

"What signs or symptoms should I watch for that might indicate a complication?"

"What is the likelihood of the scar recurring or a new scar forming after treatment?" "Do you recommend any complementary or alternative therapies alongside the primary treatment?"

Choosing the right healthcare provider is a critical step. Look for board-certified dermatologists or plastic surgeons. Board certification indicates that a physician has met rigorous standards of training, examination, and experience in their specialty.

Research their experience with scar management specifically. Do they have a particular interest or expertise in treating the type of scar you have? Reading patient reviews and testimonials can provide insights into other patients' experiences, but remember that individual results can vary.

Don't be afraid to seek a second opinion, especially for complex cases or if you have any doubts about the recommended treatment plan. A good provider will be open to discussing your concerns, will clearly explain the rationale behind their recommendations, and will involve you actively in the decision-making process. They should also be able to provide before-and-after photos of similar cases they have treated, allowing you to visualize potential outcomes.

The initial consultation is more than just an assessment; it's the beginning of a partnership. By understanding the distinct roles of dermatologists and plastic surgeons, preparing thoroughly, asking pertinent questions, and carefully selecting a qualified provider, you set yourself up for a personalized and effective scar management plan. This professional guidance, combined with your own informed participation, is the key to achieving the best possible outcomes, improving both the appearance and the quality of life impacted by your scar. Remember, achieving your scar management goals is a marathon, not a sprint, and having a trusted medical professional guiding you every step of the way significantly enhances your chances of success and ensures the process is as safe and comfortable as possible.

The journey towards optimal scar management is seldom a one-size-fits-all endeavour. While understanding your scar and setting clear goals are foundational, the true power of transformation often lies in the artful orchestration of multiple therapeutic modalities. This strategic blending of treatments, known as a multimodal approach, harnesses the synergistic capabilities of different interventions, leading to outcomes that can surpass what any single therapy could achieve in isolation.

It's about recognizing that scars, much like the skin they inhabit, are complex and dynamic entities that may benefit from a multifaceted attack.

The rationale behind combining treatments is rooted in the understanding that different therapeutic agents and procedures target distinct aspects of scar pathology. For instance, one modality might focus on reducing inflammation and redness, another on flattening raised tissue, a third on improving texture and pigment, and yet another on stimulating collagen remodelling for improved dermal structure. By layering these interventions, we can address these various components concurrently or sequentially, creating a more comprehensive and potent treatment strategy. This approach acknowledges that a single scar might present with a combination of issues – perhaps it's red and raised, or indented and discoloured – and therefore requires a multi-pronged solution to achieve the best possible aesthetic and functional improvement.

Consider the case of hypertrophic scars and keloids. These raised, often erythematous scars are characterized by an overproduction of collagen. A common and highly effective combination therapy involves the judicious use of intralesional corticosteroid injections alongside silicone-based products. Corticosteroids, when injected directly into the scar tissue, work to suppress inflammation and inhibit fibroblast proliferation, thereby reducing the thickness and height of the scar. This intervention is often potent in flattening raised lesions and alleviating associated symptoms like itching and discomfort. However, the inflammatory response can sometimes rebound, and the scar may still retain some firmness or discoloration.

This is where the concurrent or subsequent application of silicone sheeting or gel becomes invaluable. Silicone creates a semi-occlusive barrier that hydrates the scar tissue, modulates fibroblast production, and can further contribute to softening and flattening. The combined effect of reducing inflammation with corticosteroids and softening with silicone can be significantly more pronounced than using either treatment alone. For particularly stubborn or extensive keloids, a plastic surgeon might even consider excising the keloid surgically and then immediately injecting corticosteroids into the fresh wound closure, followed by a regimen of silicone sheeting at home, to prevent recurrence and promote optimal healing.

Another potent combination for managing hypertrophic and keloid scars involves the use of cryotherapy in conjunction with corticosteroid injections. Cryotherapy, which involves the application of extreme cold, can induce localized tissue damage and inflammation, leading to a reduction in fibroblast activity and collagen synthesis. When combined with intralesional corticosteroid injections, the dual mechanism of injury and anti-inflammatory action can be highly effective in reducing scar volume and improving texture. The sequence and timing of these treatments are critical, and a skilled practitioner will carefully plan this based on the scar's characteristics and the patient's response.

For atrophic scars, such as those resulting from acne or trauma, the goal is often to stimulate collagen production and improve the dermal volume and texture.

Microneedling, a minimally invasive procedure that uses fine needles to create microscopic channels in the skin, is a cornerstone therapy.

These micro-injuries trigger the skin's natural wound-healing response, leading to the production of new collagen and elastin. However, the regenerative process can be further enhanced by combining microneedling with the topical application of specific active ingredients. Immediately following microneedling, the skin's barrier is temporarily compromised, allowing for enhanced penetration of beneficial agents. For atrophic scars, serums containing growth factors, peptides, hyaluronic acid, or even low concentrations of retinoids can be applied. Growth factors can signal cells to initiate and accelerate tissue regeneration, while peptides can support collagen synthesis. Hyaluronic acid provides hydration and plumping, and retinoids can further promote collagen remodelling and cell turnover. This synergy between the physical stimulus of microneedling and the biochemical support of topical agents can lead to a more significant improvement in scar depth and surface texture than microneedling alone.

Furthermore, lasers play a pivotal role in multimodal scar management, and their application is often enhanced when combined with other therapies. Fractional ablative lasers, which create controlled thermal injury in a fractional pattern, are excellent for resurfacing the skin and stimulating collagen remodelling, particularly beneficial for depressed or textured atrophic scars. However, for scars that are also red and inflamed, a vascular laser, such as a pulsed dye laser (PDL), can be used to target and reduce the redness by collapsing the abnormal blood vessels within the scar tissue. A common strategy for scars exhibiting both textural irregularities and persistent redness is a sequential treatment protocol. A patient might first undergo a series of PDL treatments to diminish the erythema.

Once the redness has significantly subsided, fractional laser resurfacing can then be employed to address the textural issues and stimulate deeper collagen remodelling. The combination allows for a comprehensive approach, tackling both vascular and structural components of the scar.

In cases where laser therapy is employed for textural improvement, it can also be beneficially combined with microneedling. While fractional lasers ablate or create controlled heat injury, microneedling creates more mechanical disruption and can be performed at different depths. A dermatologist might recommend fractional laser treatment for deeper remodelling, followed by a course of microneedling sessions to refine the superficial texture and promote further collagen induction. The choice between or combination of these modalities depends on the specific scar characteristics, such as depth, texture, and the patient's skin type and tolerance.

Another powerful combination, particularly for scars that are not only raised but also have associated pigmentary changes (either darker or lighter than the surrounding skin), involves a phased approach. For instance, a raised, red scar might first be treated with intralesional corticosteroid injections to reduce its bulk. Once the scar has flattened significantly, subsequent treatments might involve a vascular laser to address any remaining redness, followed by a pigment-correcting laser or intense pulsed light (IPL) therapy to even out the skin tone. Alternatively, for post-inflammatory hyperpigmentation (PIH) – the dark marks left behind after a scar heals – a combination of topical agents like hydroquinone, retinoids, or azelaic acid, along with periodic IPL treatments, can be very effective in fading the discoloration.

The integration of chemical peels into a scar management plan also offers significant synergistic potential. Medium-depth chemical peels, using agents like trichloroacetic acid (TCA), can create controlled injury to the epidermis and upper dermis, promoting skin regeneration, improving texture, and helping to fade superficial discoloration. For atrophic scars, a chemical peel can be used as a standalone treatment or, more effectively, in conjunction with other modalities. For example, a series of microneedling sessions might be followed by a TCA peel to enhance overall skin resurfacing and collagen stimulation. The peel can help to further refine the skin's surface after microneedling has initiated deeper remodelling. Similarly, for scars with mild textural irregularities and PIH, a combination of a superficial peel followed by a series of microneedling treatments can yield superior results compared to either treatment performed in isolation.

The effectiveness of combining treatments is also amplified by the careful selection of patients and the precise timing of interventions. Not all scars are created equal, and a scar that is still in its active inflammatory phase might require a different initial approach than a mature, stable scar. For example, a newly formed, red, raised scar might benefit most from a combination of silicone sheeting and topical anti-inflammatory agents, with corticosteroid injections reserved for when it fails to respond.

Once the scar has matured and stabilized, then treatments focused on textural remodelling, such as laser therapy or microneedling, might become the primary focus.

Furthermore, the patient's lifestyle and commitment to home care are critical components of any successful multimodal treatment plan.

While in-office procedures address the scar directly, consistent adherence to prescribed topical treatments and sun protection at home can significantly enhance and sustain the results achieved. For example, after undergoing laser resurfacing for acne scars, a patient will likely be instructed to use specific hydrating and healing creams, along with diligent sunscreen application, to optimize the healing process and prevent

post-inflammatory hyperpigmentation. The effectiveness of a multimodal approach is therefore a collaborative effort between the healthcare provider and the patient.

The concept of combining modalities also extends to managing scars that result from different underlying causes. A surgical scar, for instance, might be managed differently than a scar from an injury or a burn. However, the principles of combining treatments often remain the same. A surgical scar that is well-approximated but slightly hypertrophic might benefit from silicone sheeting and perhaps a series of micro-needling sessions to improve its texture and colour. A burn scar, which can be extensive and involve significant changes in skin texture, colour, and even mobility, often requires a highly individualized and multi-pronged approach. This might involve a combination of laser therapy for redness and contracture, silicone therapy for softening and flattening, and potentially surgical intervention for severe contractures.

When considering a multimodal approach, it is crucial to have realistic expectations. While combining therapies can lead to remarkable improvements, complete scar eradication is often not achievable. The goal is typically to make the scar less noticeable, improve its texture and colour, and restore any lost function.

A qualified dermatologist or plastic surgeon will carefully assess your scar, discuss your personal goals, and propose a treatment plan that optimally combines modalities to achieve the best possible outcome for your specific situation. They will explain the rationale behind each suggested treatment, the expected timeline, potential side effects, and the anticipated results. This collaborative discussion ensures that you are an active participant in your scar management journey, empowered to make informed decisions about your treatment pathway. The true art of scar management lies not in a single miracle cure, but in the intelligent and tailored combination of available tools to sculpt a more harmonious and less conspicuous result.

Navigating the financial landscape of scar treatment is a crucial step in any personalized management plan. While the desire for smoother, less noticeable skin is paramount, understanding the associated costs and the intricacies of insurance coverage is equally important for making informed decisions and ensuring the long-term feasibility of your treatment journey.

This section aims to demystify the financial aspects, providing a realistic overview of expenses, explaining the difference between cosmetic and medically necessary procedures, and offering practical advice on budgeting and insurance navigation.

The cost of scar treatments can vary dramatically, influenced by the type and severity of the scar, the chosen treatment modalities, the geographic location of the provider, and the practitioner's expertise.

At the most accessible end of the spectrum are over-the-counter (OTC) products.

These can range from simple silicone sheets and gels, which might cost anywhere from $20 to $100 or more per product, to topical scar creams containing ingredients like onion extract, vitamin E, or retinoids, priced typically between $30 and $80. While these are generally affordable, their effectiveness is often limited to milder scars and may require consistent, long-term application to see subtle improvements. For individuals with more significant scarring, these products serve more as complementary adjuncts to more intensive treatments rather than standalone solutions.

Moving into the realm of professional interventions, the costs escalate considerably. Minor procedures performed in a dermatologist's or plastic surgeon's office, such as topical or intralesional corticosteroid injections, can range from $100 to $500 per session, depending on the number of lesions treated and the complexity of the injection. Chemical peels, a common treatment for superficial discoloration and texture improvement, can cost between $150 and $600 per session, with deeper peels naturally commanding higher prices. The number of sessions required for noticeable results can range from one to several, significantly impacting the overall expenditure.

Laser therapies represent a significant investment. Different types of lasers carry different price points, and the total cost is often determined by the size of the treatment area and the number of sessions needed. For instance, fractional laser resurfacing, often used for atrophic acne scars or surgical scars, can cost anywhere from $500 to $2,000 or more per session. Vascular lasers, used to target redness in hypertrophic or keloid scars, might fall within a similar range. The total treatment plan for laser therapy could easily run into several thousand dollars, especially if multiple sessions are required for optimal outcomes.

More invasive procedures, such as microneedling with radiofrequency (RF) or platelet-rich plasma (PRP) add-ons, can further increase the cost.

A single session of microneedling might range from $300 to $700, while RF microneedling, which combines skin needling with radiofrequency energy to enhance collagen stimulation, could be between $600 and $1,200 per session.

When considering multiple sessions of these advanced treatments, the cumulative cost can be substantial.

Surgical scar revision, which involves excising and re-suturing a scar or performing more complex reconstructive techniques, represents the highest end of the cost spectrum.

These procedures can range from $1,000 for a minor revision to $10,000 or more for extensive reconstructions, especially if they are performed under general anaesthesia or require specialized techniques.

The surgeon's fees, anaesthesia costs, and facility fees all contribute to the overall expense of surgical interventions.

Given these costs, understanding insurance coverage is paramount.

The distinction between a "medically necessary" procedure and a "cosmetic" procedure is the primary determinant of whether insurance will provide any reimbursement.

Generally, insurance plans consider treatments medically necessary if they are performed to correct a functional impairment or to alleviate significant pain, itching, or discomfort directly related to the scar.

For example, a scar that restricts movement (a functional impairment) or causes chronic pain or severe itching might be considered for coverage.

Conversely, treatments aimed solely at improving the aesthetic appearance of a scar, even if the scar is prominent or distressing to the individual, are often classified as cosmetic and will not be covered by insurance.

This distinction can be nuanced and often depends on the specific wording of your insurance policy and the justification provided by your healthcare provider.

Navigating insurance claims for scar treatment requires diligence and persistence. The first step is to thoroughly review your insurance policy or speak with a representative to understand what is covered. When consulting with your dermatologist or plastic surgeon, it is crucial to discuss whether your scar might qualify as medically necessary. If it does, your provider will typically need to submit a detailed letter of medical necessity to your insurance company, outlining the functional limitations or symptoms caused by the scar and explaining how the proposed treatment will address these issues. This letter should include diagnostic codes that support the medical necessity claim.

It is also important to be aware that even if a procedure is deemed medically necessary, there may still be out-of-pocket expenses. Deductibles, co-payments, and co-insurance will apply according to your plan.

Some insurance plans may have limitations on the number of treatments covered per year or may require pre-authorization for specific procedures. It is essential to obtain pre-authorization whenever possible to avoid unexpected denials of coverage.

When a scar is the result of an injury or accident covered by workers' compensation or a personal injury claim, the situation changes.

In such cases, the cost of scar treatment might be covered by the responsible party's insurance. However, this typically requires proper documentation of the injury and a clear link between the injury and the need for scar revision.

For treatments that are definitively cosmetic, budgeting becomes even more critical. It is advisable to obtain detailed cost estimates from your healthcare provider for the entire recommended treatment plan, not just a single session. This should include all anticipated fees: surgeon's fee, anaesthesia fee, facility fee, and any post-operative care or prescription costs. Don't hesitate to ask for a breakdown of these costs.

Once you have a clear understanding of the total expense, you can explore various payment options. Many medical practices offer in-house financing plans which often provide interest-free periods for qualified applicants. Exploring these options can make larger treatment plans more manageable by allowing you to spread payments over several months or even years.

Another effective budgeting strategy is to prioritize treatments. If the full recommended plan is financially out of reach, discuss with your provider which interventions would yield the most significant improvement if undertaken first. A phased approach, where you tackle the most impactful treatments initially and then gradually work through others as your budget allows, can be a practical way to achieve your goals over time.

It is also wise to factor in potential hidden costs. This could include transportation to and from appointments, time off work for recovery (which might mean lost wages), and any prescription medications or specialized skincare products recommended post-treatment.

Building a small contingency fund into your overall budget can help buffer against unforeseen expenses.

When discussing costs with your provider, be open about your financial concerns. A reputable practice will be understanding and may be able to suggest alternative treatments that are more budget-friendly while still addressing your primary concerns. They might also be able to provide information on whether specific treatments have historically been covered by insurance for similar conditions, even if coverage is not guaranteed.

Ultimately, informed financial planning is as vital to successful scar management as the chosen treatments themselves. By understanding the potential costs, clearly distinguishing between medically necessary and cosmetic procedures, diligently navigating insurance policies, and exploring flexible payment options, you can create a realistic and achievable budget that supports your journey toward scar improvement without causing undue financial strain. This proactive approach ensures that your focus can remain on healing and achieving the best possible outcome for your skin.

The journey toward scar improvement is a dynamic process, and while achieving significant aesthetic and functional results is a monumental accomplishment, the commitment to long-term scar maintenance and prevention is equally critical. This phase moves beyond active treatment to a sustainable regimen that preserves the gains made and safeguards against future scarring. It is about cultivating a lifelong habit of mindful skin care, ensuring that the progress achieved is not only maintained but that your skin remains resilient and healthy.

One of the cornerstones of long-term scar maintenance is **unwavering sun protection**. Scars, particularly those that are still maturing (typically within the first 1-2 years post-injury or surgery), are more susceptible to hyperpigmentation and photodamage. The melanin in scar tissue is often more sensitive to ultraviolet (UV) radiation. Exposure to the sun without adequate protection can lead to a darkening of the scar, making it more noticeable and potentially permanent. This darkening, known as post-inflammatory hyperpigmentation, can be notoriously difficult to treat. Therefore, a diligent daily application of broad-spectrum sunscreen with an SPF of 30 or higher is non-negotiable. This should be applied to all scar sites, even on cloudy days, as UV rays can penetrate cloud cover. Furthermore, when spending extended periods outdoors, consider physical barriers such as wide-brimmed hats, protective clothing, and seeking shade during peak sun hours (typically between 10 am and 4 pm). This consistent vigilance against the sun's harmful rays is perhaps the single most effective strategy for preventing discoloration and maintaining the scar's improved appearance.

Beyond sun protection, the **consistent use of recommended topical agents** plays a vital role in ongoing scar care. While the intensive phase of treatment might involve a cocktail of prescription-strength retinoids, silicone sheeting, or specialized serums, the maintenance phase often involves a more streamlined yet equally important application. Many individuals find that continuing with silicone gel or sheets, even after significant scar flattening, can help maintain hydration and pliability.

This can prevent the scar from becoming dry, itchy, or developing a raised, firm texture again.

Similarly, periodic use of over-the-counter scar creams containing ingredients like onion extract, centella asiatica, or vitamin E can offer continued nourishment and support skin barrier function. The key here is adherence; even if the scar looks good, a few minutes dedicated each day or several times a week to applying these supportive topicals can prevent subtle changes that might otherwise go unnoticed until they become more problematic.

It's about reinforcing the skin's healing capacity and keeping it in its optimal state. Your dermatologist or plastic surgeon will likely provide specific recommendations for maintenance topicals based on the type of scar you had and the treatments you underwent. It's important to follow these tailored guidelines, understanding that these products are not just for active treatment but for sustained well-being.

Adherence to any **prescribed follow-up care** is another crucial element of long-term scar management. While some scars may require only a few post-treatment check-ups, others, particularly those that were more severe or complex, might benefit from longer-term monitoring. These follow-up appointments, whether with your dermatologist, plastic surgeon, or even a wound care specialist, serve several vital purposes. Firstly, they allow your healthcare provider to monitor the scar's evolution, ensuring that no adverse reactions or new issues are developing. Secondly, they provide an opportunity to adjust your maintenance regimen as needed. For instance, if initial maintenance topicals become less effective or if new environmental factors impact the scar, your provider can update your plan. Thirdly, these appointments offer a chance to address any lingering concerns you might have.

Seeing a professional periodically reinforces the understanding that scar care is an ongoing commitment, not a one-time fix. It ensures that you remain informed and empowered in managing your skin health.

A significant aspect of long-term scar management involves **preventing new scarring from future injuries**. This proactive approach is essential for anyone who has experienced scarring, as it underscores the importance of meticulous wound care. When a new injury occurs – be it a cut, scrape, burn, or even a minor surgical procedure – the way it is managed in the initial stages can dramatically influence the outcome in terms of scarring.

The principles of good wound care are consistent: **cleanliness, moisture balance, and protection**.

Upon sustaining a new wound, the immediate priority is to clean it thoroughly. Gentle cleansing with mild soap and water is usually sufficient for superficial injuries. For deeper wounds, it is important to seek medical attention to ensure proper cleaning and assessment for any foreign bodies or underlying damage. Avoiding harsh antiseptics like hydrogen peroxide or alcohol, which can damage delicate healing tissues, is generally recommended unless specifically advised by a healthcare professional.

Maintaining a **moist wound environment** is paramount for optimal healing and minimizing scar formation. Contrary to older beliefs that wounds should be kept dry, modern wound care principles emphasize the benefits of a moist environment. This can be achieved through the use of sterile dressings, hydrocolloid bandages, or even simple applications of petroleum jelly or a specialized wound gel.

A moist environment promotes cell migration, reduces inflammation, and helps prevent the formation of hard, dry scabs that can impede healing and contribute to thicker scars. Applying a thin layer of antibiotic ointment or petroleum jelly and covering the wound with a non-stick sterile dressing is often recommended for minor cuts and abrasions. For more significant wounds, your healthcare provider might recommend advanced wound dressings that create and maintain this optimal moist environment.

**Protecting the healing wound** from external factors is equally important. This involves shielding it from further trauma, contamination, and excessive moisture (from external sources, not the wound itself). For wounds that are prone to tension, such as those on joints or areas of high movement, strategies to reduce tension can be beneficial.

This might include using flexible bandages that allow for some movement without stressing the wound edges, or in some cases, temporary immobilization.

Furthermore, understanding the **risk factors associated with new scarring** can inform preventative measures. Individuals who are genetically predisposed to keloid or hypertrophic scarring, or those with darker skin tones who are more prone to post-inflammatory hyperpigmentation, may need to be particularly vigilant.

For these individuals, even minor injuries require careful management. If a new wound occurs in an area that previously scarred poorly, it is wise to consult with your dermatologist or plastic surgeon early on.

They can recommend specific preventative treatments, such as the application of silicone sheeting or topical corticosteroids to the healing wound, to minimize the likelihood of unfavourable scarring from the outset.

The impact of **infection** on scar formation cannot be overstated. Any wound that becomes infected is far more likely to result in significant scarring. Signs of infection include increased redness, warmth, swelling, pus formation, and fever. If any of these symptoms are present, prompt medical attention is crucial to treat the infection and minimize its impact on healing and scarring.

In cases of burns, specific wound care protocols are essential. Gentle cleansing, the application of specialized burn ointments, and appropriate dressing techniques are vital to promote healing and reduce scar formation. For larger or deeper burns, professional medical care is always necessary to prevent infection and optimize healing.

When it comes to surgical incisions, while the surgeon's technique plays a significant role in minimizing scarring, diligent **post-operative care** by the patient is also critical. This often involves keeping the incision clean and dry as instructed, using any prescribed topical treatments, and avoiding activities that could put tension on the sutures. Once sutures are removed or the wound has closed, transitioning to scar maintenance therapies like silicone sheeting and sunscreen becomes paramount.

Ultimately, cultivating a mindset of **proactive skin health and continuous scar care** empowers individuals to manage their skin effectively throughout their lives.

This involves understanding that scars, while often permanent, can be managed and their appearance significantly improved.

It means embracing a consistent, long-term approach that prioritizes sun protection, utilizes beneficial topical agents, adheres to professional guidance, and applies meticulous care to any new injuries.

By integrating these strategies into your daily routine, you not only preserve the results of your past treatments but also build resilience against future scarring, fostering confidence and a lasting sense of well-being in your skin.

This proactive and informed approach ensures that the journey towards scar improvement is not just a chapter, but a continuous narrative of healthy, well-cared-for skin.

# DEFINITIONS

**Atrophic Scar:** A scar that is depressed below the surrounding skin, often appearing thin, wrinkled, or pitted. Examples include acne scars and stretch marks.

**Collagen:** A structural protein that provides strength and elasticity to the skin and other connective tissues. Scar tissue is primarily composed of collagen.

**Dermis:** The layer of skin beneath the epidermis, containing connective tissue, hair follicles, sweat glands, and blood vessels. Most scar formation occurs in the dermis.

**Epidermis:** The outermost layer of the skin.

**Fibroblast:** A type of cell found in connective tissue that produces collagen and other fibers. Fibroblasts play a crucial role in wound healing and scar formation.

**Granulation Tissue:** New connective tissue and blood vessels formed on the surface of a wound during the healing process.

**Hypertrophic Scar:** A raised, red, and often itchy scar that remains within the boundaries of the original wound.

**Inflammation:** The body's natural response to injury or infection, characterized by redness, swelling, heat, and pain. It is a critical phase of wound healing but can also contribute to scar formation if prolonged.

**Keloid:** An overgrowth of scar tissue that extends beyond the original wound boundaries. Keloids are often firm, rubbery, and can be itchy or painful.

**Macrophage:** A type of white blood cell that engulfs and digests cellular debris, foreign substances, microbes, cancer cells, and anything else that does not have the type of proteins specific to healthy bodily cells on its surface. They are important in the inflammatory phase of wound healing.

**Melanocyte:** A cell responsible for producing melanin, the pigment that gives skin its color. Melanin plays a role in post-inflammatory hyperpigmentation of scars.

**Platelet:** A small blood cell that plays a key role in blood clotting and wound healing by releasing growth factors.

**Post-inflammatory Hyperpigmentation (PIH):** Darkening of the skin that occurs after an inflammatory process, such as an injury or acne.

**Scar Maturation:** The final stage of wound healing where the scar tissue remodels, flattens, and becomes less red and more pliable over time.

**Tension:** The pulling force across a wound. High tension can lead to wider and more prominent scars.

**Wound Dehiscence:** The splitting open of a wound.

Made in the USA
Las Vegas, NV
04 November 2026

57464471R00107